A Tooth from the Tiger's Mouth

HOW TO TREAT YOUR INJURIES
WITH POWERFUL HEALING SECRETS
OF THE GREAT CHINESE WARRIORS

TOM BISIO

Illustrations by Xue Zhu

ATRIA PAPERBACK

New York London Toronto Sydney New Delhi

An Imprint of Simon & Schuster, Inc.
1230 Avenue of the Americas
New York, NY 10020

This Atria Paperback edition January 2020

ATRIA PAPERBACK and colophon are trademarks of Simon & Schuster, Inc.

For information about special discounts for bulk purchases, please contact Simon & Schuster Special Sales at 1-866-506-1949 or business@simonandschuster.com.

The Simon & Schuster Speakers Bureau can bring authors to your live event. For more information or to book an event, contact the Simon & Schuster Speakers Bureau at 1-866-248-3049 or visit our website at www.simonspeakers.com.

Manufactured in the United States of America

19 20 18

The Library of Congress has cataloged the Fireside edition as follows:

Bisio, Tom.
A tooth from the tiger's mouth : how to treat your injuries with powerful healing secrets of the great Chinese warriors / Tom Bisio.
p. cm.
"A Fireside book."
Includes index.
1. Sports medicine. 2. Medicine, Chinese. 3. Sports injuries—Alternative treatment.
I. Title.
RC1210.B57 2004
617.1'027—dc22 2004049590

ISBN 978-0-7432-4551-7
ISBN 978-1-4391-8877-4 (ebook)

A Tooth from
the Tiger's Mouth

To Vince Black

for his selfless teaching, inspiration, and friendship.

ACKNOWLEDGMENTS

My thanks to Mary Evans, for her weekly refrain of "Where is my book proposal?" Without her patience and encouragement, this book would not have been written.

I want to thank Valerie Ghent for her enthusiasm and help, for listening to my ideas tumble out and helping to put them into coherent sentences. And Val, as always, thank you for your technical assistance with computer snafus.

I would like to acknowledge my colleagues at 5th St. Acupuncture for their support and their forbearance in listening to me talk about the book.

Many thanks to Huang Guo-qi, who has helped me in countless ways over many years. He helped make possible the illustrations in this book.

My thanks to Xue Zhu for her wonderful drawings.

Thanks to my son Virgil, who put up with my pleas of "just one more sentence" when it was time to play basketball.

Thank you, Caroline Sutton, for guiding me through all the steps of publishing a book.

My heartfelt thanks to my parents, Attilio and Rosemary, for their love.

And thanks to Sweetpea, who curled up on my papers and kept me company as I wrote.

CONTENTS

Part I: Principles of Chinese Sports Medicine

Part II: Injury Prevention: Exercise, Diet, and Health Preservation

Part III: The Therapies of Chinese Sports Medicine

Part IV: Treatments for Common Sports Injuries and Miscellaneous Injuries

PART I

Principles of Chinese Sports Medicine

INTRODUCTION TO PART I

When I began to study martial arts some thirty years ago, I never imagined that practicing the fighting arts would lead me so far into the study of medicine. My inspiration to train hard in those early years came from stories of unbeatable masters, Asian knight-errants who defeated all comers and helped the weak and downtrodden. In time, I studied a variety of fighting disciplines under a number of different masters, became a professional martial arts instructor, and fought in full-contact matches in places as far apart as New York's Chinatown and the Philippines.

Somewhere along the way, I found myself drawn to the stories of teachers whose superlative fighting skills were tempered by their ability to heal the sick and injured. During my earlier training, I met many great fighters, but few healers. However, like most subcultures, the martial arts world is small. If you look hard enough, you will find what you are searching for. Then it is merely a matter of having the courage or, in my case, the naive temerity to seize the chance. To make a long story short, I met the right teacher at the right time, and he set my feet on the path—an evening of being bounced off the walls of a hotel room, followed by an animated discussion of the connection between the martial arts and Chinese medicine that went into the wee hours, did the trick.

To my obsession with the martial arts I added apprenticeships in herbology and kung fu medicine, three years of acupuncture school, and endless study of books on Chinese medicine. Gradually I became familiar with the many facets of Chinese medicine.

I began to treat patients and later opened a clinic. There are many specialties in Chinese medicine, but the kung fu medicine that evolved into Chinese sports medicine has always excited me the most. One reason for my enthusiasm is that Chinese sports medicine uses all the therapies available in Chinese medicine—herbology, acupuncture, and moxibustion, physical therapy and exercise, massage, and even diet therapy—allowing treatments to be more easily adapted to each injury and, more important, each individual. Another is that its often miraculous effectiveness satisfies my own impatience to see quick results.

My experience is that the West tends to view Chinese medicine as either an exotic Eastern philosophy with little practical value or a kind of quaint folk medicine that sometimes achieves inexplicable results but is full of poetic imagery that is confusing to the uninitiated. "Scientific" is not normally a word associated with Chinese medicine. Yet Chinese medicine *is* a science, based upon acute observations of the natural world and man's place in that world. These are not the observations of one man or one woman or the viewpoint of a small cult of true believers. These observations were not made in a decade or over the course of one or two centuries. They are the result of two millennia of research, scholarship, debate, and practical experience by millions of people. The result is an elegant, sophisticated system of medicine that is clinically effective.

Sports medicine is one area in which Chinese medicine is particularly effective, but despite the explosion of books on alternative health and Eastern medicine, little has been written on the subject. Previous books have listed some of the herbal remedies employed in Chinese medicine or delineated treatments for specific injuries, but until now, no book has explained how to simply and practically use this medicine to treat an injury from the moment it occurs until you return to the playing field.

In medicine, receiving the right treatment at the right time makes all the difference. Nowhere is this more true than with sports, where correct treatment can prevent a minor injury from becoming a chronic problem. This book was born out of many things—the urgings of friends and students as well as the debt I owe my teachers to pass on their knowledge, but mostly it was born out of my frustration at seeing so many people who would not need to be in my office if they had treated their injuries correctly from the moment they occurred. This book is my attempt to make Chinese sports medicine available to everyone so they can get back to doing the activities they love as soon as possible. I hope it makes a difference.

I still get my inspiration from the stories of the old masters. These stories and the pictures of my teachers on the wall of my clinic serve as daily reminders of the long and diverse lineages linking the twin disciplines of fighting and healing. In the East, the masters of today are always considered inferior to the great masters of the past. While this sentiment keeps the teacher's or doctor's ego in check and offsets the praise of devoted students and satisfied patients, it is not merely a device to keep us humble. The feats of the past masters remind us of the vast experience and accumulated knowledge that form the foundation of Chinese medicine and breathe life into its practice.

CHAPTER 1

A Tooth from the Tiger's Mouth
Martial Origins, Modern Alternative

China, 1899. The empress dowager sits on the imperial throne. Flood and famine devastate the countryside. Antiforeign sentiment grows, and the lives of European diplomats are threatened by fanatical martial arts societies. The country is on the brink of the Boxer Rebellion. Amid this turmoil, two men, one from the north and one from the south, both martial arts warriors and healers, became legends.

Sun Lu-tang was one of the most famous boxers of the northern *nei jia,* or "internal," school of martial arts. By the time of the Boxer Rebellion, he had already studied with some of the most famous martial arts masters in China. Tales of his encounters with bandits and his effortless victories in challenge matches with rival masters still inspire today's generation of kung fu enthusiasts.

Some of the most compelling stories about Sun revolve around his compassion for those injured in combat and his ability to heal them. On one occasion, he defeated a group of bandits and then resuscitated them and set their dislocated bones. Another time, a large, powerful student attempted to injure the diminutive Sun. Sun lightly struck an acupuncture point on the student's arm, incapacitating him. The next day the arm had turned black. Sun administered an herbal remedy, and the student recovered with a humbler attitude. Sun was not familiar just with acupuncture and herbal medicine, he also practiced Taoist health exercises reputed to harmonize the functioning of the internal organs. Sun attributed his robust health in old age to these exercises. Even in his seventies, traversing the steep mountain paths of northern China, he was able to outpace students decades younger.

Wong Fei-hung, Sun's counterpart in southern China, developed a reputation as a peerless fighter and skilled physician. His exploits are today immortalized in the films of Jet Li. Wong initially learned kung fu from his father, one of the famed "Ten Tigers of Guandong" (the ten top martial artists in southern China). His father passed on to Wong many of the secrets of the fighting monks from southern Shaolin. When his father was challenged by a rival master, the thirteen-year-old Wong took his place, easily defeating the challenger. He later studied with other great masters in southern China. His many exploits in helping the common Chinese people made him famous by the early twentieth century. Wong founded a clinic known as Po Chi Lam ("Precious Iris Woods," a reference to his skill with herbal medicine). At Po Chi Lam he taught martial arts and the related medical skills of acupuncture, herbal medicine, and bone-setting. Wong's fighting system, the "Hung Fist," still flourishes today, and his herbal recipes are still used to treat training injuries.

Fighting skill and the physician's art seem like odd bedfellows, yet in China they have been linked for nearly two millennia. The skills exhibited by Sun Lu-tang and Wong Fei-hung were the distillation of centuries of warfare and civil strife. Martial arts medicine was an outgrowth of warfare. Treatment of battlefield injuries had to be simple and effective, so that soldiers could return to combat as quickly as possible. In armies composed of martial arts adepts, even training for warfare could be incredibly brutal. Dislocated joints and broken bones were not unusual and sprains and contusions commonplace. Over centuries, martial arts masters, Shaolin monks, and Taoist recluses developed hundreds of herbal formulas that could treat everything from spear wounds to fractured ribs.

Military commanders were also accomplished martial artists

and often well versed in practical medical skills. Marshal Yue Fei, China's renowned military leader in the twelfth century, studied all the warrior arts, including traditional medicine. The effectiveness of Yue Fei's troops is attributed to their rigorous training in the martial arts, and Yue Fei himself is credited with the creation of several unique kung fu styles as well as the Eight Brocade Plus exercises presented later in this book.

Looking at the past from our modern perspective, we could easily assume that without antibiotics and today's surgical wizardry, people died from even minor wounds. In fact, this was much more the case during America's Civil War than in conflicts in China. The ancient Chinese employed hundreds of herbal substances that could kill pain, stop infection, reduce inflammation and swelling, and help tissue regenerate. Some of Wong Fei-hung's medical knowledge originated in India, where ancient texts describe Hindu physicians performing many surgical operations, such as cesarean section, hernia operations, and rhinoplasty. In AD 927, two physicians successfully trepanned the skull of a Hindu king, using a general anesthetic. Merchants, pilgrims, Buddhist monks, and soldiers traveling the Silk Road brought Indian medicine and fighting traditions to China. Ta Mo, a Buddhist teacher from India, noticed that during meditation many of the students were so frail that they fell asleep. He created a series of exercises to strengthen the body. Later, Ta Mo's "18 Luohan" exercises became the basis of the Shaolin fighting arts. These traditions were exemplified by Hua Tuo, perhaps the most famous doctor of the Han dynasty (206 BC–AD 220). Hua Tuo performed surgeries using herbal anesthetics. A student of Taoist mountain sages, he also developed a regime of health exercises based on the movements of animals and derived from martial arts traditions.

By the Tang dynasty, China had a rich tradition of medicine based on practical experience. Although physicians had to be well versed in both Chinese and Buddhist medical texts, they were above all clinicians who prided themselves on getting results. The Shaolin temple became a repository for much of this knowledge. Martial arts medicine was one of Shaolin's closely guarded secrets, passed down by oral tradition. With the destruction of the Shaolin temple in the Qing dynasty, the monks fled and spread their knowledge to martial arts societies throughout southern China and Southeast Asia.

At the time of the Boxer Rebellion, the separation of martial arts from military science had begun. Guns and cannon replaced traditional weapons and martial ways. Men like Sun Lu-tang and Wong Fei-hung were part of the last generation directly connected to the old ways. During their lifetime, martial arts and their attendant medical traditions passed from arts of war to arts of self-defense and self-cultivation. Competitive martial arts schools replaced warring armies. Schools with effective methods guarded them jealously from other schools. Challenges and even outright brawls between schools were rampant. Martial arts teachers kept knowledge from their own students, often passing on herbal formulas and other techniques to only one or two worthy disciples. Even today, many kung fu schools use a liniment to treat strains and sprains called die da jiu (literally "hit-fall wine"), whose formula is kept secret from even the most advanced and loyal students.

In the twentieth century, this secrecy and the push toward industrialization combined to ensure that fewer and fewer people had the medical knowledge of men like Sun and Wong. Traditional teachings that had withstood the test of centuries were gradually eroded. A more crippling blow was China's Cultural Revolution. During that time, the teaching of martial arts and traditional medicine was suppressed, making it dangerous to admit knowledge of either one. Many of the great teachers of martial arts were killed, and the Shaolin monks were all but wiped out of existence. As fewer people were instructed in these methods, martial arts medicine became more secretive and esoteric. Later, traditional medicine came back into favor. Acupuncture and herbal medicine regained their former popularity, but the medicine of the martial arts that today we call Chinese sports medicine remained a closely guarded secret, protected by an older generation of martial arts masters out of favor with the Chinese government. Consequently, Chinese sports medicine is not taught even in colleges of traditional Chinese medicine. In the United States today, acupuncture schools proliferate, yet Chinese sports medicine is absent from the curriculum. Add to this the emphasis in these schools on internal medicine, and the result is that the majority of their graduates don't know how to treat sprains, contusions, and other musculoskeletal injuries. Despite this state of affairs, the medical skills of Wong Fei-hung and Sun Lu-tang are not lost. They have been kept alive by people like me: modern practitioners of Chinese sports medicine who learned their craft in traditional schools of martial arts.

The medical feats of Sun Lu-tang and Wong Fei-hung are not just the stuff of stories. Many injuries can be treated easily and cheaply with knowledge of a few basic principles and readily available herbal formulas. Although I have studied at modern acupuncture schools and today run a busy clinic specializing in athletic injuries, the most effective treatments I know come out of thirty years of study and research in the ancient martial arts traditions. Like Sun Lu-tang, I treated an arm that turned black from a martial arts strike. A simple poultice of san huang san ("three yellow powder"), one of the formulas covered in this book, resolved the problem in two days. I have treated nonhealing fractures that mystified doctors using formerly secret Shaolin formulas that aid the knitting of broken bones. I have seen countless sprained ankles heal in a fraction of the usual time using Chinese sports medicine. Western medicine can offer little help for these types of injuries. I was not a licensed practitioner of Chinese medicine when I first treated these injuries. I was a martial arts instructor with a rudimentary knowledge of Chinese sports medicine. With this book in your hands, you will have at your fingertips far more information than I had.

Chinese sports medicine has always been like the Chinese saying "a tooth from the tiger's mouth": knowledge difficult and even dangerous to obtain. It has survived centuries of change and upheaval because it works. The goal of every athlete and every active person in every time and place has been to get back to the activities they love as soon as possible. In our busy modern world, this has never been more true. This book can help you do this.

HOW TO USE THIS BOOK

Presumably, most authors arrange their books to be read from start to finish, each chapter building on the previous one. This book is designed to be read that way, but with an understanding that many of you will want to skip to the part that concerns you and perhaps browse through other sections of interest. With that in mind, the book is divided into four parts. Part 1 presents the theoretical background of treating sports injuries: the anatomy of injury, the basic principles of using Chinese medicine to treat them, and the basic dos and don'ts of Chinese sports medicine.

Parts 2 and 3 present the four pillars of Chinese sports medicine, the therapies passed down by the secret martial arts societies in China:

1. External Herb Therapy

The secret injury formulas of the Chinese martial arts that stimulate local circulation, kill pain, and promote healing in the injured tissues. These formulas have never before been shared with the general public. (See chapters 10–12.)

2. Internal Herb Therapy

Herbal teas, pills, and tinctures that reduce inflammation and strengthen the body's ability to heal itself. The herbal formulas used to heal tendon and ligament injuries and the specific herbs that help broken bones to heal. (See chapter 15.)

3. Physical Medicine

Treatment methods that directly manipulate, stimulate, or heat the injured area, such as cupping (chapter 9), acupressure (chapter 13), self-massage (chapter 14), and moxibustion (chapter 16), to break up the accumulations of stagnant fluids and blood that can lead to chronic pain and dysfunction. These methods are all easily self-administered and can be applied by anyone.

4. Health Preservation

The closely guarded training methods of martial arts masters that enhance athletic performance, prevent injury, and preserve health.

Also dietary secrets of the Chinese martial arts and the foods that can aid or prevent injuries from healing. (See chapters 5, 6, and 7.) I anticipate that many of you will skip right to part 4. Here the most common sports injuries and their appropriate treatment are arranged in alphabetical order. Try to read the earlier chapters or at least go back to them, especially those in part 1, so that you are familiar with the basic concepts on which the therapies are based. As much as possible, related information is either repeated in different sections of the book or cross-referenced to the relevant chapter to keep you from having to hunt through the whole book to find an herbal formula or specific treatment.

CHAPTER 2

Sports Injuries East and West

MODERN MEDICINE AND
TRADITIONAL CHINESE MEDICINE

There is no such thing as perfect health. The very concept of perfect health is an illusion. For many of us, health means feeling no pain or weakness. In fact, health is a balancing act, a constant series of small shifts back and forth to maintain a general sense of equilibrium. For this reason, when the body moves out of balance, medical interventions must be chosen carefully, with the goal of returning the body to a balanced state.

In the West, illness, weakness, or pain is perceived as "not good," and steps are taken to rectify the situation. Interventions in modern medicine often take the form of painkillers, anti-inflammatories, antibiotics, antidepressants, or surgery. These interventions may lead to a change in symptoms. These new symptoms, in their turn, may also require correction. Each shift may be seen as a separate entity and each set of symptoms as a different disease or syndrome. Each is a disease to be overcome and defeated. As diseases and syndromes proliferate and the technology used to treat them grows more complex, specialization becomes a necessity. The very nature of specialization in modern medicine requires that the specialist work within the borders of his or her understanding, often without regard for the whole. The patient's sense of his or her own body and the interconnectedness of the whole is overridden by the expertise of the specialist, who is concerned with only one part.

As new discoveries and advances are made, old wisdoms are regarded as outdated and are discarded. While this seems to make sense, in fact it can lead to further confusion. What was perceived as "good" at one point in time is now "bad." These changes can come so fast that we forget they occurred. When I was growing up, butter was considered a major culprit in heart disease and margarine was eaten by every family I knew. More recent studies indicate that margarine is far worse for one's arteries than butter, but a whole generation ate margarine for twenty years. Public perception of what is healthy shifts with each new study that comes out, even when the new study contradicts the previous one. Even more recently in the news is the discovery that women who take hormone supplements after menopause increase their risk of developing dementia, heart disease, and certain types of cancer. In this case, using drugs to "turn back the clock" worked against the body's inner rhythms and its innate wisdom. Millions of women took hormones to prevent hot flashes and osteoporosis, problems that Chinese medicine has treated for centuries with diet and exercise and herbal supplements.

Modern medicine is very good at understanding disease but does not give us the tools to understand health. It cannot offer clear-cut ideas about what health is because it has no standard to go by. Traditional Chinese medicine, on the other hand, has an understanding of health that dates back to one of its oldest books, the *Huang Ti Nei Jing, The Yellow Emperor's Classic of Internal Medicine* (third century BC). These ideas have never become outdated despite the technological advances of Western medicine. Why? Because in ancient times, the Chinese observed the minute changes that occurred in the human body in relation to season, weather, climate, diet, exercise, and emotional shifts. From these observations was born a system of medicine that perceived the fundamental holism of the human organism and its interconnectedness with the surrounding environment. Thus Chinese medicine offers a unique perspective on maintaining a state of harmonious balance in the human body.

Modern medicine has a tendency to view as normal dysfunctions that stem from an unhealthy lifestyle. If the average fifty-year-old has some arthritis in his knees, this is considered normal. He is told to take anti-inflammatories or painkillers and he goes back to jogging. By masking the pain in this way, further damage is often done. If the knee is too bothersome, a knee replacement is always an option. Viewing average health as "normal" combined with the intensive specialization of the modern physician has led modern medicine to a philosophical approach akin to that of a high-level mechanic. Parts wear out and are jury-rigged or replaced. Each patient is not so much an individual as an identical model that will undergo exactly the same procedure for the same problem.

Another view is that our body is built to last a lifetime if we treat it right, that each individual has a different amount of vital energy, and that it is this vital energy that often determines how different bodies will react to different diseases and how quickly we will recover. Chinese medicine is based upon the concept of qi (vital energy), and it is qi more than any other single idea that led the Chinese to embrace a very different philosophy of medicine from what developed in the West. Ancient Chinese physicians focused their treatments not only on dispelling illness, but also on harmonizing and nurturing the qi of their patients. This led Chinese medicine to hold up as its standard individuals who were healthy into old age because they led harmonious and balanced lives. Thus the Chinese developed principles of medicine based on high standards of health as well as physical and mental performance. Traditionally, health preservation through correct living was considered to be the highest form of medicine. Intervention by a medical practitioner in the form of herbs, drugs, or physical medicine was kept to a minimum to restore the patient to balance with the least possible side effects, and physicians felt they had failed if a patient became seriously ill.

Just thinking this way offers a profound alternative. If we live right and use medical knowledge appropriately and intelligently, we can lead healthy, active lives even into old age. One of my most unforgettable memories from China is the large number of elderly people up in the morning exercising, demonstrating levels of flexibility and strength that we normally associate with much younger athletes.

Chinese medicine employs methods that are not injurious to the patient by attempting to harmonize the body's natural functions and stimulate its innate ability to heal. These methods are not mystical or esoteric, they are based on a commonsense approach to diagnosis and treatment. A famous martial arts teacher in New York's Chinatown once asked, "If common sense is so common, how come so few people have it?" Often we neglect our common sense when we are fearful and in pain, and we rush to take pills or elect surgery as a first-choice treatment. This is not common sense when there are other alternatives. Taking drugs to cure one problem and cause another does not make much sense, yet people do it every day. It is common sense to see the body as an interconnected whole. Cutting-edge research by Western medical doctors if anything confirms this viewpoint that is one of the cornerstones of Chinese medicine, yet people are told every day that their chronic shoulder injury has nothing to do with their hip pain. My patients are constantly amazed when I confirm their own feeling that two problems in different areas of the body can be connected. This confirmation of their own bodily felt sense of connection is invaluable for them to understand how imbalances occur and how to heal and prevent them.

The tendency to view a medical model as an objective reality, rather than a means of describing what is happening in a moment in time inside a living being, can lead to many mistakes, including intolerance to alternative approaches. Both Western and Eastern medicine have different strengths and weaknesses. The approach that best serves the patient is to use strengths of each whenever possible. To this end, the reader is advised to consult a Western-trained medical doctor for an initial diagnosis. In the case of sports medicine, this is particularly important when there is a question about the severity of an injury. The diagnostic procedures of Western medicine are very useful in helping the athlete decide which type of medicine is most appropriate to the situation and, if serious injury is ruled out, may give him or her more confidence and precision in employing the Eastern approach.

ANATOMY OF AN INJURY—EAST AND WEST

An ankle sprain serves as the perfect model to begin this comparison and to examine injuries and how they heal. Not only is an ankle sprain one of the most common sports injuries, it can happen just crossing the street. Anyone who has had a badly sprained ankle knows how painful it can be. Ankle sprains can be slow to heal and often prevent or interfere with athletic activities for a long time afterward. Many of the principles used to treat sprained ankles apply to other joint, tendon, and muscle injuries.

When you sprain an ankle, there is usually a tearing, wrenching sensation, followed almost immediately by pain and weakness. Ankle sprains most often occur because the foot is tipped inward so that the body weight falls on the outside edge of the foot, straining or spraining the ligaments on the outside of the ankle. Sometimes the pain dissipates in a minute or two and the ankle seems okay, only to swell and become more painful over the next twenty to thirty minutes. Sprains are usually considered ligament injuries. Ligaments are made up of fibrous connective tissue connecting bone to bone. Ligaments help maintain the integrity of the joint. However, in most sprains muscles and tendons are injured as well.

LIGAMENTS: Fibrous connective tissue connecting bone to bone. Ligaments are instrumental in maintaining joint integrity.

TENDONS: Fibrous connective tissue found at the ends of muscle, connecting muscle to bone.

MUSCLES: Contractile connective tissue that has the ability to contract or shorten, pulling on tendons to create movement.

Sprains and most muscle and tendon injuries are usually classified by their degree of severity.

GRADE 1 SPRAIN: Stretching of a few fibers with minimal tearing of those fibers.

GRADE 2 SPRAIN: Partial tearing of fibers. Often a hole or a slight dent can be felt in the fibers.

GRADE 3 SPRAIN: Extensive or complete rupture. Grade 3 sprains also include tearing a tendon or ligament off the bone.

When a sprain occurs there is usually inflammation. Blood flows into the injured area, and it swells with blood and tissue fluids. The result is the injured area feels hot to the touch, and there is local redness, swelling, and pain. The redness and sensation of heat are caused by the dilation of arterioles and other small blood vessels as well as greater vascular permeability, which serve to increase the amount of blood brought to the local area. Blood and fluids back up in the tissues, causing swelling. The blood brings with it white blood cells in order to clean up dead tissue and fight possible infection. Nutrient building blocks are also brought to the local area, where they attempt to initiate the healing process and rebuild damaged tissue. Most of the initial swelling is actually blood from broken blood vessels that lace the soft tissue around the joint. As ligaments and tendons stretch and tear, blood from ruptured blood vessels becomes trapped in the local tissues. Inflammation is an important part of the healing process. It is also the body's attempt to "splint" the injury, thereby protecting it from further trauma. The problem is that this splinting with blood and fluids blocks normal circulation and prevents movement. It also causes tissues that were not normally in contact with one another to rub together. This can lead to further inflammation and irritation.

One other complication common to sprains is that bones can be slightly displaced. In ankle sprains, the talus bone will often move out of its normal alignment as tendons and ligaments are stretched. Sometimes it will not seat evenly again when it snaps back. It will then remain slightly out of alignment, often undetected by X-rays and MRIs, causing continued pain and weakness in the ankle even after the inflammation is gone.

With sprains, strains, and even fractures it is important to reduce swelling as quickly as possible so that further irritation and inflammation can be prevented and rehabilitation can begin. Most people are familiar with how thin a broken arm or leg looks when the cast comes off after six weeks. What they don't realize is that muscle atrophy begins after only a few days of restricted movement. The less atrophy that occurs, the less weakness there will be later. It is often this weakness that prevents the athlete from returning to a sport and sets him or her up for reinjury. This can become a vicious cycle of chronic inflammation, atrophy, pain, weakness, and repeated injury.

By moving the body, and therefore the muscles, tendons, and ligaments, we significantly reduce joint stiffness and weakness. Movement also increases blood circulation through injured tissue and back to the heart, clearing away dead cells and reducing swelling, thereby allowing healing to occur. Additionally, movement, stretching, and strength training correct muscle imbalances that may have made the area more vulnerable to injury.

The Western treatment for reducing this kind of inflammation is known as "RICE": rest, ice, compression, and elevation. It is usually recommended that RICE begin in the first twenty-four hours after the injury.

Rest is obvious. Continued activity may further inflame and irritate the injury.

Ice contracts the blood vessels in the local area, reducing swelling. It reduces pain and cools the heat of the inflammation. In Western medicine, ice is universally recommended for all kinds of inflammation, including that present in chronic injuries. In Chinese medicine, it is almost never used and is considered a culprit in joint injuries that don't heal properly, because cold causes contraction of the muscles and tends to freeze and congeal the fluids that cause swelling, ultimately preventing their complete reabsorption.

Compression limits swelling. Usually an elastic bandage is wrapped around the injured area to compress the tissues, thereby limiting blood flow into the area. This is contrary to Chinese medicine, where such constriction is felt to cause blood to stagnate and congeal above and below the injury. This slows reabsorption into the blood vessels.

Elevation involves simply raising the injured part above the level of the heart to let the force of gravity aid in draining excess fluid. This method is also employed in Chinese sports medicine.

Once inflammation and swelling are reduced, treatment is directed at restoring movement and circulation to the injured area through gentle movement and exercise. Sometimes after the first twenty-four to forty-eight hours of RICE, when the swelling has stabilized, contrast baths (alternating hot and cold baths) are recommended. Contrast baths cause an alternating contraction and dilation of blood vessels in the local area, which serves to pump blood and fluids through the injured tissue. This helps restore normal circulation to the local area.

This mechanical approach that Western medicine uses to diagnose and treat ankle sprains is useful and in many ways similar to Chinese medicine, but beyond RICE, it does not give the athlete many tools to work with in rehabilitating an injury, and it leaves many questions unanswered:

Why do some sprains heal while others do not?

Why does one athlete quickly shake off an injury and return to his or her sport while another athlete with the same injury is caught in a cycle of chronic pain and reinjury?

Why do some fractures and sprains hurt more in damp or cold weather?

Why do some injuries become arthritic in later life while others do not?

Fortunately, Chinese medicine provides clear, concise answers to these kinds of questions and offers a host of treatments for different injuries.

At first glance, it appears that Chinese medicine's approach to examining a sports injury such as an ankle sprain is not all that different from that of Western medicine. An impact or force acts on the body, disrupting the flow of qi (vital energy) and blood in the local area. This force can take many forms. It can be the twisting, wrenching force common to a sprain, a compressive force as in a fall or impact, or the whiplash force of tissues stretching and snapping back. If the force is great enough, it may affect distant areas of the body as well.

Blood and qi stagnate in the local area, blocking circulation and causing swelling and pain. The profound consequences of this

Ice Is for Dead People

In 1984, I trained in Taiwan with Hsu Hong-chi, my teacher's teacher in Xing-Yi kung fu. Known locally as "Magic Hands" because of his skill in setting bones, Master Hsu was one of those rare teachers whose incredible skills are enhanced by his wisdom and humor.

One day after training I watched as he treated a fellow student with an ankle sprain. When I mentioned the idea of using ice to reduce the swelling, he responded with the simple statement "Ice is for dead people." I remember being taken aback by this blunt offhand remark, yet it reflects the commonsense approach of Chinese medicine.

Ice is very useful for preserving things in a static state. It slows or halts the decay of food and dead bodies but does not help damaged tissue repair itself. Ice does reduce the initial swelling and inflammation of a fresh injury, and it does reduce pain, but at a cost. Contracting local blood vessels and tissues by freezing them inhibits the restoration of normal circulation. The static blood and fluids congeal, contract, and harden with icing, making them harder or impossible to disperse later. It is not uncommon to see a sprained ankle that was iced still slightly swollen more than a year after the original injury.

Cold causes contraction of the muscles. When you go out on a cold day, the muscles contract automatically to produce warmth. You can feel how the body literally draws into itself when exposed to the cold. Every athlete knows that it is harder to stretch and easier to pull a muscle in cold weather. Icing an injured area causes further contraction in muscles, ligaments, and tendons that are already contracted in reaction to being overstretched. This further slows the natural healing process and prevents the return of normal movement.

In Chinese medicine, there is an idea that cold and damp can penetrate areas of the body where the vital energy has been compromised.

simple idea become apparent if the relationship of qi and blood is understood.

Qi is the vital force or, for lack of a better word in English, the energy responsible for all movement in the body. The circulation

---

This can lead to an arthritic type of pain that often increases with weather changes and is difficult to treat. I still rue the day I iced my fractured patella. It has taken years of treatment to prevent it from hurting in cold and rainy weather.

So why is ice used so extensively? It is a mystery to me, especially when you consider that Chinese sports medicine offers five alternatives that, when used together, reduce swelling and inflammation and restore normal circulation quickly, without any of the unwanted effects produced by icing:

1. Emergency acupoints to move energy, kill pain, and stimulate circulation. (See chapter 13.)

2. Cupping and bleeding the local area to actually draw out and disperse blood and fluid that is coagulating and blocking normal circulation. Often this reduces pain immediately. (See chapter 9.).

3. Self-massage with liniments such as trauma liniment that move the blood, reduce inflammation, and kill pain. This helps to remove static fluids and blood from the area, reducing swelling. (See chapter 10.)

4. Energetically cooling herbal poultices and plasters that reduce inflammation but also stimulate circulation and help torn muscles and tendons to heal. (See chapter 11.)

5. Herbal pills or powders that are taken orally to promote blood circulation and prevent blood from stagnating further. (See chapter 15.)

If you must use ice, or if nothing else is available, try to apply it for only ten minutes out of every hour. This will help reduce the swelling but minimize the negative side effects.

of blood in the blood vessels and of fluid through the tissues, respiration, the complex processes of digestion, the release and production of hormones, cellular activity, all are dependent on the body's internal energy, or qi.

Qi flows in a capillarylike network through the skin and the flesh, the muscles and the tendons. It brings blood and fluids to these tissues, nourishing and moistening them so that the skin and the flesh shine with vitality and the muscles and tendons contract and move in a smooth, coordinated fashion. Qi also warms the body's exterior and controls the opening and closing of the pores, aiding the body in adapting to temperature changes.

The relationship of qi and blood is summed up as follows: "Qi is the commander of the blood, and blood is the mother of qi." This means that blood cannot move without the driving action of the qi, and in turn, the organs that produce and nurture the qi are dependent on the nourishment of the blood in order to function. This is not as esoteric as it sounds. The lungs and the heart oxygenate the blood so that oxygen is carried to the organ and every cell in the body. There is a direct relationship between oxygen consumption and energy and heat production in the body. The organs of digestion such as the spleen, pancreas, stomach, and intestines break down food and liquids and transform food into sugars like glucose that provide the fuel for skeletal muscle. These unconscious metabolic activities are visible manifestations of the unseen vital force. The implications of this arrangement go further: qi is constantly coalescing and transforming into blood, and in turn, blood transforms into qi. They are like two sides of the same coin.

Although in the more superficial layers of the body qi travels in a network of tiny vessels, deeper in the body it travels in more discrete pathways called "meridians" that connect with the internal organs, sensory organs, and the brain. In an injury such as a sprain or strain, qi is blocked, but sometimes only at the superficial level of the skin, flesh, and muscles. This results in pain and stiffness. There may be little or no bruising, meaning that few blood vessels were ruptured and blood circulation is not significantly impaired. There is often slight swelling or palpable lumps under the skin and a sensation of heat (inflammation). Swelling is the result of the stagnation of qi (and therefore the blood and fluids it moves), its normal movement disrupted by the impact or force. The stagnation of qi acts like a dam. Blood and fluids back up behind the dam, causing swelling or lumps. The sensation of heat is due to the warming action of the qi overheating the local area as qi backs up and accumulates.

The impulse to rub an injured area is a natural, unconscious attempt to push the circulation through the area, breaking the dam and therefore restoring a free flow of energy, blood, and fluid and reducing the pain. Pain is considered to be a result of stagnation—a lack of free flow of qi and blood—in the injured area. The concept of pain in Chinese sports medicine is succinctly explained in the following equation:

Pain = lack of free flow of qi (stagnation)

If an injury is more severe, more blood vessels are broken and there may be structural damage, such as torn muscles and ligaments or broken bones. The disruption of normal circulation is greater, and more qi and blood stagnate behind this larger dam. There is more swelling because there is greater stagnation of blood and fluids. The injured area is hotter to the touch as more qi accumulates, bringing with it more blood and fluids. In a bad sprain there is usually visible bruising that appears fairly soon after the injury.

Stagnant blood tends to lodge in the spaces between layers of tissue. As it congeals, it glues these tissues together, creating adhesions. Layers of tissue that formerly slid smoothly across one another now stick and catch so that they interfere with normal functioning. This restricts movement and causes pain.

If stagnant blood and fluids are not cleared and normal circulation restored, the injured area has less vital energy than before. It becomes a kind of "dead zone" that never feels quite right. Even after the swelling and inflammation are gone, it takes more of the body's energy than normal to push circulation through or around the area. Over time the area becomes sensitive to cold or damp weather, in part because of diminished circulation. It may occasionally swell or feel numb. The pain can return or increase when the body's energy is depleted or when you are overtired, under stress, or have the flu.

When an injury develops to this point, it is called "*bi* syndrome." *Bi* refers to a chronic obstruction of energy in a joint or muscle. This chronic obstruction can be due to the exposure of an already weakened area to a cold and damp climate or to repeated exposures to cold and damp, which overcomes the body's attempts to warm and protect itself. With modern technology, cold and damp can be artificially induced. I have treated several people who worked in refrigerators or freezers who developed arthritic problems in a relatively short period of time.

It is easy to try to dismiss these ideas as unscientific, yet millions of people who take painkillers suffer from discomfort that returns or worsens with weather changes. Many of the fur trappers of our American West suffered from arthritis in their legs that they attributed to wading in icy mountain streams to set beaver traps. In Europe today there is still an awareness of the deleterious effects of cold drafts.

Bi syndrome often occurs in joints, where the thick fibrous tissue that makes up the joint capsule can prevent circulation to the interior part of the capsule. This inner layer of the joint capsule is composed of cartilage, which has no direct blood supply. This is why a torn meniscus (the cartilage of the knee) takes so long to heal. However, *bi* syndrome can also occur in the muscles. I remember a woman who ran the New York City Marathon inappropriately dressed for a day that turned unexpectedly cold and wet. By the end of the race her legs became heavy, painful, and numb. This condition persisted for weeks afterward. Her muscles felt cold to the touch and were quite tight and painful. Cold and damp weather changes made the condition worse. The use of warming liniments, moxibustion (heating the injured area by burning herbs over acupoints), and herbal formulas that helped to move the blood and warm the legs restored normal circulation and drove out the cold. She is still running today.

To heal properly, damaged tissue must regenerate. That is, it must be replaced with healthy, functional tissue. If normal circulation is not restored and the body does not have the energy and the nutrients to do this, the tissue cannot repair itself. Adhesions form, limiting movement and causing low-level inflammation. In cases where there is repeated reinjury and chronic inflammation, normal tissue can be replaced with thick fibrous tissue or scar tissue. Continued inflammation can cause calcium to be deposited in the muscles, tendons, and joints, creating more inflammation, thereby perpetuating the cycle. This is not uncommon with bursitis of the shoulder or Achilles' tendonitis.

In looking at this progression from acute to chronic injury, you can understand the importance of treating minor injuries as soon as possible to prevent them from developing into chronic obstructions. It is all too easy to dismiss a bruise or sprain as "nothing" (a mistake I have made many times). If treated right away, it really will be nothing and you can simply focus on playing your sport.

TO HEAL OR NOT TO HEAL

Why do some injuries linger and become chronic while others just disappear with a little rest? The idea of vital energy is dismissed as unscientific in Western medicine, yet we talk about people having a "strong constitution" and therefore healing faster or being more resistant to illness. The same treatment will not make all patients better, and they will not all heal at the same rate if they have different amounts of vital energy. Obviously, if an injury is severe enough, with large amounts of structural damage, it will be difficult to restore normal functioning, but very often injuries do not heal because the qi or vital energy is in some way compromised. There are many ways this can happen. Stress is one of the biggest factors. There is a good reason Europeans (at least those who could afford it) have a tradition of residing at a sanitarium or spa to recuperate from a serious illness or an injury. Getting plenty of rest and fresh air, eating good food, and living stress-free allow a large portion of the body's resources to be directed toward repairing the injured tissue.

In modern life, we barely give ourselves a rest. We return immediately to a stressful job or lifestyle. Even after major surgery, people often feel pressured to return to work as soon as possible. Added to this are meals eaten on the run and the consumption of processed food or junk food. This combination exhausts the body and starves it of nutrients. The body is left with too few resources, and what resources it has are being allocated to keep up with the fast-paced world around us.

Age is also a factor in healing. Young people have a surplus of vital energy. Even if stressed and overworked, they have enough extra to help them recover quickly. Young children are a good example of this. They are bursting with energy, always in motion, running, jumping, and climbing. Although in some ways they are more fragile than adults, they heal more quickly and bounce back from injuries that would cripple grown-ups. Their bones and muscles are pliable, and they are in many ways less susceptible to injury. This is in part due to their surplus of vital energy.

Taking the time to let the body heal is difficult. We want to get back to our sport or activity as soon as possible. Once the pain is gone, we try to take up right where we left off. I remember talking to one of my patients who had almost become a professional tennis player but decided on a career in music instead. I asked him if he still played an occasional game. He shook his head no and explained that he had tried to but always injured himself. His body remembered what it was like to play at a high level, but it was no longer as strong as when he had played every day. It was not prepared for the sudden stresses put on it by a single game of tennis. This is exactly what happens when you return to a sport after an injury or layoff.

In the case of a sprained ankle, although you are ready to play at the level you played before, your ankle is not. The overstretched ligaments need time to return to normal. A general rule is that as the pain subsides, movement should increase. This means increasing the range of motion as the swelling decreases. The next phase is to walk unaided without a limp. Strength and flexibility exercises are added gradually. Start slow and gradually increase the intensity when the sport or activity is resumed. Therapy and rehabilitation exercise should be continued until there is no further pain *while playing*. If the pain persists, it is important to consult a medical professional.

HEALTHY ORGANS/HEALTHY TISSUES

For muscles, tendons, ligaments, and bones to be healthy, they must be adequately supplied with blood, moistened by fluids, and provided nutrients. The tissues are therefore dependent on the organs that produce, circulate, and supply these substances. In Chinese medicine, the internal organs are seen not just as physical structures, but as the hubs of a whole web of functional interactions taking place on many levels and throughout the entire body. Viewed in this way, impaired functioning of the internal organs can have profound consequences on associated tissues. Three of these connections are of particular importance in sports medicine:

LIVER: sinews (tendon, ligament, cartilage).

SPLEEN: flesh/muscles.

KIDNEY: bones.

The liver is connected to the sinews. The term *sinews* refers to several kinds of soft tissue that connect muscle to bone and bone to bone. These are tendons and ligaments and the articular cartilage and fibrous connective tissue of the joint capsule. In Chinese medicine, the liver is considered to be responsible for smooth coordinated movement of the body and for the unimpeded movement of energy through the meridian network. The liver receives and extracts newly absorbed nutrients, which are then released according to the physical demands placed upon the body. Vast amounts of blood pass through the liver (1.5 liters, almost a third of the heart's output, passes through the liver each minute), carrying nutrients to the tissues. The Chinese say that it is the blood of the liver that nourishes the sinews. When tendons and ligaments are overstretched or torn, herbs that tonify the liver blood are prescribed to help these tissues heal properly.

The spleen and the stomach connect with the muscle bellies and the flesh. These organs oversee a whole network of processes, including the breakdown of food and drink and the absorption of nutrients. When the spleen and stomach function correctly, nutrients are made available to fuel physical activity and to nourish the other internal organs. When they are not functioning properly, the limbs feel heavy and weak and the muscles lose tonus. Herbs that tonify the qi can aid the spleen and the stomach's ability to nourish and supply energy to the muscles, but eating properly is the best way to ensure that the spleen and stomach function correctly (see chapter 7).

It must be understood that when the Chinese refer to the spleen, they are not referring to the organ only. In Chinese medicine, the spleen includes the organ and a web of interconnections that include the actions of the pancreas and the organs of digestion. In addition, the spleen is considered to work with the kidneys and the lungs to circulate and regulate fluids.

The kidneys are said to "rule the bones." They contribute to the production of the bone marrow, which in turn helps to produce healthy bones. The relationship of the kidneys and the bones is well-known in modern medicine. For example, when the supply of oxygen is less than the demand, the kidneys produce a substance called "erythropoietin," which is released into the blood, where it travels to the bone marrow; there it stimulates the production of red blood cells. Interestingly, many of the herbs that help to heal fractures, and which strengthen tendons and bones, are kidney- and liver-tonifying herbs (see chapter 4).

These relationships help to explain why muscles, tendons, ligaments, and bones sometimes fail to heal properly or completely. Sometimes the final stage in the treatment of a sports injury involves the tonification or harmonizing of one of these organ systems. Although some organ-harmonizing methods will be discussed in this book, they may require consultation with a licensed acupuncturist or herbalist. The importance of these relationships should not be underestimated. If you are not getting better weeks or months after an injury, it may be because an internal imbalance is preventing the body from directing its full attention to healing the injury. I remember a patient with knee pain who had undergone successful treatment with chemotherapy for a lymphoma earlier in the year. X-rays and an MRI found no structural abnormalities. Acupuncture and massage had done little more than temporarily relieve the pain. He did not make a connection between his knee pain and the chemotherapy. The muscles of his legs were flaccid, and he felt weak and tired. The chemotherapy had weakened the blood and depleted his vital energy. His body had no reserves left to heal the strained knee. I stimulated acupoints that energized the body and the legs by heating them using moxibustion (chapter 16). These points also strengthen the functioning of the spleen and liver. This, combined with herbs to strengthen the qi and the blood, helped him to recover and resume exercise.

There are even more profound implications to this relationship of the organs and tissues. *Damage to the tissues can actually affect the functioning of the internal organs.* Although I had learned that this was possible from my teachers, in clinical practice it is often hard to see a direct link between an injury to a tendon or ligament and an organ dysfunction that may occur years later. I gave lip service to this idea until I treated a middle-aged woman with a decade-old ankle injury that had never healed properly. She also mentioned that she had to get up to urinate six or seven times a night, a more recent problem that had developed in the last two years. On the first treatment I focused on her ankle, thinking I would address the bladder problem later. I used acupuncture, massage, and gentle manipulation to realign the ankle joint. By the end of the treatment, her ankle was pain-free. She said she felt her foot was "on straight" for the first time in years. When she returned the following week, she said her bladder was fine and she could sleep through the night without urinating. I was amazed, but what had happened was very clear. Her bladder problem came from her ankle. The bladder meridian travels through the outside of the ankle. It was exactly this meridian that had been twisted when she injured her ankle. Over a period of years, damage to the bladder meridian had begun to affect the functioning of the bladder itself. This experience graphically illustrates how properly treating minor injuries can prevent more serious problems from manifesting later.

RECOVERY TIMES

One of the first questions an injured athlete asks is, "How long until I can start training again?" In the previous discussion, I mentioned several factors that can influence healing time. Different people heal at different rates, and different tissues also have different healing times. This is in part due to the amount of blood supplied to those tissues by the circulatory system. Blood brings with it nutrient building blocks that repair damaged tissue as well as the oxygen necessary to produce heat and energy.

The following healing times are approximations based on healthy individuals who are receiving adequate rest and nutrition. They can be considerably longer in those who are more depleted, suffering from chronic disease, or not receiving adequate rest and nutrition. If you have had surgery, be prepared for a longer recovery time than your orthopedist tells you. Recovery times for sports injuries are often based on the experiences of professional or Olympic athletes, who have the luxury to focus their whole being on recovery, often assisted by a team of physical therapists, massage therapists, and acupuncturists. If you work all day and squeeze in your rehabilitation work between dinner and putting the kids to bed, recovery may take longer.

Muscles

Muscles heal fast because they are filled with blood vessels. Pulled muscles are really tears in muscle tissue. The small blood vessels that run throughout muscle tissue are torn as well. That is why muscle pulls are often accompanied by a black-and-blue discoloration at the site of the injury. Pulled muscles usually take about three weeks to heal. Healing time will be longer if there is extensive tearing or if the muscle is reinjured before it is fully healed.

Bones

Bones also heal relatively quickly. They have a large blood supply, and blood cells are formed within the bone marrow. In a healthy person, a simple fracture will usually heal in five to six weeks. For greater detail on fractures and bone healing, see chapter 4.

Ligaments and Tendons (Sinews)

Ligaments and tendons are composed of thicker fibrous tissue. Unlike the muscles, they do not have a large direct supply of blood. When damaged, they heal more slowly than bones or muscles, often taking six to eight weeks. If tendons or ligaments are severely torn or overstretched, they can take considerably longer to heal or may never heal completely without intervention.

Cartilage and Discs

Although related to ligaments and tendons, according to Chinese medicine, spinal discs and cartilage can take considerably longer to heal. Three to six months is a realistic estimate. If treated properly at the outset, they have a greater chance of healing properly. Repeated damage to these structures will make them harder to heal. In cases where there is extensive damage to cartilage and discs, surgery may be required. In these cases, Chinese sports medicine can be used to speed recovery and postsurgical healing.

How to Examine an Injury

PAIN

Pain is usually the first sign that something is wrong. For purposes of self-evaluation, it is useful to divide pain into three categories:

- MILD PAIN: Often disappears with activity and does not prevent one from performing exercise or participating in a sport. It is not uncommon for the pain of the early stage of tendonitis to lessen or disappear completely with activity. When an injury has just occurred, the pain may be quite severe for a minute or two and then lighten up and disappear altogether over the next several minutes. Usually this type of pain does not keep you awake at night. Often massage and the application of liniments before and after activity is enough to keep this kind of pain from becoming worse. If mild pain is chronic, it may be worth getting a diagnosis to help you decide which treatments may be effective.

- MODERATE PAIN: Does not prevent sleep but can impede performance and does not disappear with activity. Sometimes this kind of pain starts out mild and increases over time, gradually inhibiting performance. Chronic groin and hamstring pulls or slightly sprained ankles and wrists can fall into this category. If the injured area becomes twisted during sleep, it can wake you. It is not uncommon with wrist injuries for the wrist to become twisted under the body during sleep, thereby aggravating the injury. Sleeping with a wrist brace or skateboarding wrist guard can help.

- SEVERE PAIN: Stops activity and is not stopped by mild over-the-counter painkillers. It interrupts sleep and if bad enough may make you feel nauseated. The injury should be immediately examined by a physician. This type of pain often accompanies bone breaks or torn tendons and ligaments.

- RADIATING PAIN: Pain that radiates to another area or down the leg or arm. Often this means there is impingement of some structure on a nerve, causing a radiating pain. The impingement may be from muscular tension creating pressure on the nerve or from a more direct pressure such as protrusion of a disc on one of the spinal nerves. Often sciatica is caused by tension in the back muscles or the piriformis muscle, which lies under the large muscles of the buttocks. Radiating pain can be serious, so it is worth having a professional examine you to find out what is going on. Be aware that an MRI may not always reveal the source of the problem and that many people have bulging discs but do not experience any pain.

Pain is to some degree a cultural phenomenon. Different cultures and different people have a different relationship to pain. What one person experiences as excruciating may be shrugged off by another. This is particularly true with children who sometimes react strongly to minor pain and then return to play a few minutes later. On the other hand, some children will uncomplainingly return to the game with severe injuries but may be limping or not using the injured part.

Pain is not always by itself a clear indicator of the severity of an injury. I remember my son woke from sleep crying with severe pain in the area of his collarbone. It was extremely tender to the touch and had all the symptoms of a fracture, although there was no swelling and no obvious break could be felt. As he had fallen the day before, I could not rule out the possibility of a hairline fracture. A visit to the emergency room for X-rays showed nothing. It turned out to be a very painful muscle strain, which let up slowly over the next day or so. Contrast this with a friend's son, who was brought to me after a fall and did not complain of any pain. It turned out that he had a broken collarbone.

VISUAL INSPECTION

Deformity

Look for obvious deformity.

- It is often useful to compare one side of the body with the other to see if bony landmarks, joint creases, and muscles match up or to see if one side is more swollen. Have the landmarks shifted on the injured side, or are they symmetrical with the uninjured side? Marked deformity accompanied by pain is a good indication of a serious problem. Don't risk moving the injured part; immobilize it and get professional help as soon as possible.

- Try to find out exactly where it hurts. Sometimes X-rays do not reveal obvious differences that can be seen with the naked eye. A kickboxer with pain in his hand from punching his opponent in a match showed me a hand with a metacarpal bone clearly protruding. X-rays showed nothing, yet hitting the bag was painful. We treated it as a subluxation (a bone partially displaced), and he was able to go back to training.

Bruising

Bruising is a sign of ruptured blood vessels in the local area. There may be a large black-and-blue spot accompanied by swelling or just a subtle discoloration. Chinese sports medicine categorizes bruises according to their color.

1. BLACK: Bruising is down to the level of the bone. Keep in mind, though, that sometimes bone bruises can be felt but not seen.

2. GREEN: Bruising is down to the level of the tendon.

3. YELLOW: Bruising is more superficial, at the level of the muscle. There can be considerable overlap among these colors. For example, pulled muscles are accompanied by greenish yellow bruises.

Swelling

Swelling indicates stagnation of fluid and/or blood and the possible presence of inflammation. Different kinds of swelling may indicate different things.

1. PITTING SWELLING: A swollen area that has depressions in it, especially after applying slight pressure. This can indicate a deeper level of swelling often associated with fractures or severe sprains, although people who are retaining water because of internal imbalances may also have pitting swelling or edema.

2. SWELLING THAT PUSHES OUTWARD IN A CONTAINED AREA: Common in sprains where blood and fluids from ruptured blood vessels have accumulated in the local area.

3. HOT, RED SWELLING: Indicates inflammation and accumulation of fluids and qi. This kind of swelling requires the application of liniments (chapter 10) or poultices and plasters (chapter 11) that have a cooling, anti-inflammatory effect.

4. COTTONLIKE SWELLING: Looks mushy or cottony and often feels that way to the touch. This often indicates a fracture and should be X-rayed.

Body symmetry

Look at the symmetry of the two sides of the body to see if more global imbalances may be causing or contributing to a problem.

- Look at relative shoulder and hip heights. A raised hip may indicate that your back is tighter on one side, which can contribute to ankle, knee, and hip problems.

- Do your knees roughly line up with the shinbone and the ankle, or do they fall inward or outward? Do your ankles fall inward (inversion) or outward (eversion)? Knees that fall outward may indicate an imbalance in the muscles of the thigh. The muscles on the outside of the leg may be much stronger and tighter than those on the inside of the leg.

- Is the range of motion equal on both sides of the body, or is one side more restricted, and with what specific movements?

TOUCH

Touch the injured area gently and lightly, and gradually go deeper. Even if there is a fracture, gentle pressure will not do any harm. Be careful if there is an obvious deformity or a lot of swelling.

- If you can squeeze and press an area of bone without finding a specific area of tenderness, there is probably not a fracture. If there is a specific area of tenderness on the bone with persistent swelling, it may be fractured.

- If the area feels hot to the touch and is swollen, there is probably inflammation.

- If it feels cold to the touch, it means there is reduced circulation in the local area. Check carefully. Sometimes the surface skin level feels warm, but as you palpate deeper there is a feeling of cold.

MOVEMENT

- In cases of massive severe swelling and deformity after an injury, immobilize the injured part and seek medical help.

- Does pain increase or decrease with movement?

- What kinds of movements help or hurt? For example, in the case of muscles does it hurt more to contract the muscle or to stretch it? Torn or pulled muscles often hurt worse when stretched, because stretching puts tension on the torn muscle fibers.

- Check the range of motion and compare the injured side with the uninjured side. If you know what movements help or aggravate the problem, you can see what structures (muscles, bones, and so on) are affected.

- Sometimes with joint injuries, certain movements elicit a popping, cracking noise. If you move and touch the area at the same time, you may feel that something slips or clunks in one part of the range of motion. Many people who experience this automatically assume they have arthritis. Tendons and muscles work along a track, and around joints in particular, they often thread their way through narrow grooves in the bone. Through injury or improper use, they can slip out of the groove and come off the track and then slip back in again. This is particularly common in the shoulder area, where the joint is held in place primarily by the tendons of the muscles that make up the rotator cuff. Treatment usually involves gentle manipulation and corrective exercises.

SUMMARY

Whatever your injury, whether it be minor or so severe that it requires hospitalization, Chinese sports medicine advocates immediate treatment. Treat minor problems promptly and they are less likely to develop into larger problems or chronic conditions.

CHAPTER 3

Sprains, Strains, and Pain
The Three Stages of
Healing Sinew Injuries

Sinew injuries are not only the most common type of sports injury, they also plague many of us who don't play sports but perform repetitive tasks like typing at the computer or gardening. Sinews are the complex connections of soft tissue that surround the joints. Muscles, tendons, and ligaments encased in fibrous connective tissue hold the joints together. When a joint is subjected to the types of stresses imposed upon it by sports activities, these tissues bear the brunt of the strain. In Chinese medicine, these connective tissues around the joint are collectively referred to as *jin. Jin* is often translated as "sinews," a concept that includes tendons, ligaments, cartilage, and the fibrous connective tissue around the joint capsule. Interestingly, modern medicine recognizes that during early fetal development all of these tissues develop from one layer of cells called the "mesoderm."

As we saw in chapter 2, sinew injuries are categorized according to their severity. In a mild strain or sprain, the sinews are stretched abruptly, creating microscopic tears in tendons and ligaments. In severe sprains, complete tears may occur, creating instability of the joint. If there is only minor swelling and the joint can still function without pain, then the injury is probably minor. With correct treatment, the microscopic tears will heal fairly quickly and full use is often resumed within a week. Inability to use the joint or to support the body (if the sprain is in the lower limb), accompanied by dark blue or black swelling, indicates a more severe injury that may require an MRI or X-rays.

Chinese sports medicine recognizes that there are three distinct stages in the healing of sinew injuries:

STAGE 1—ACUTE

This stage starts from the moment the injury occurs and usually lasts from one to seven days. It is characterized by swelling, redness, and pain and possibly a local sensation of heat, indicating inflammation. If the trauma is minor, this stage may last only two to three days. If the injury is more severe, it may be a full week before swelling, redness, and pain begin to subside. The swelling is the result of the stagnation of qi (vital energy) and blood and body fluids because their normal movement has been disrupted by the force of the injury. This causes blood to accumulate outside the blood vessels in the soft tissue, creating a dark blue or black swelling.

Principles of Treatment

- Restore normal circulation to the injured area by reducing swelling, stimulating local circulation, and reducing the redness and heat associated with inflammation.

- Restore the flow of qi and blood in order to reduce pain and allow the joint to regain its mobility. Remember, in Chinese medicine pain equals the lack of free flow of qi, blood, and fluids.

- Use movement and exercise to strengthen the injured area in order to prevent reinjury and to further improve circulation. Movement that stimulates local circulation without overstressing damaged tissue can actually help reduce pain and swelling.

• At this stage *avoid* local applications of heat, hot compresses, soaks, heating pads, and hot tubs. Adding heat to an already inflamed joint can be like throwing gasoline on a fire. It can easily result in more swelling and pain, thereby delaying the healing process. Warming therapies are useful in stage 2, when the initial inflammation and swelling are gone.

Treatment

1. **San huang san** (chapter 11): San huang san is the single most useful herbal formula that can be applied to a severe injury during the acute stage. If you do nothing else, san huang san alone can produce amazing results. Even if the sprain is severe, you can apply san huang san before going to the doctor to reduce the swelling and inflammation. San huang san is composed of cooling herbs that reduce inflammation while breaking up blood stasis. This is the start of restoring free flow of blood and qi. It is the main substitute for ice, which also reduces inflammation but can create further stasis by constricting blood vessels and congealing stagnant fluids. If san huang san is not available, trauma liniment (chapter 10) or plasters such as yunnan paiyao plaster or Wu Yang pain-relieving plaster (chapter 11) may be used instead.

2. **Bleeding and cupping** (chapter 9): Bleeding the injured area with a sterile lancet, followed by cupping (creating a vacuum inside a glass cup, thereby producing a drawing effect on the local area), directly removes stagnant blood and fluids from the injured area. This "breaks" the beaver dam, reestablishing the free flow of qi and blood. I am constantly amazed at how quickly and significantly this ancient "folk medicine" technique can reduce pain and swelling. Cupping can be followed by a few minutes of massage and then a poultice of san huang san to increase the effectiveness of the treatment.

3. **Acupressure and massage** (chapters 13 and 14): Pressure on acupoints such as stomach 36 (an important point for leg

Analogy of a Beaver Dam

The blockage of qi, blood, and fluids that accompanies sprains and strains is much like a beaver dam. The initial obstruction caused by the force of the injury acts like the sticks, mud, and leaves of the dam. The free-flowing clear, cool water of the mountain stream is slowed down and reduced to a trickle as stagnant water backs up behind the dam. In the same way that the still water heats up in the sun, stagnant fluids in our body are heated up by our naturally warm temperature, creating local heat and inflammation. Just as the water behind the beaver dam becomes cloudy as sediment is deposited there, so too in the human body nutrients and white blood cells rush to the injured area and accumulate.

Applying heat dilates blood vessels, bringing more circulation and more fluids to the injured area and resulting in a bigger pond behind the dam. This can create more swelling and inflammation. The solution is to remove the dam while encouraging the stagnant water behind it to move freely again, reestablishing the natural movement of the stream.

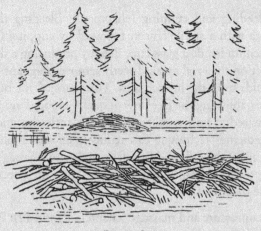

Figure 1.

pain), combined with gentle massage above and below the point of injury, helps encourage the movement and reabsorption of stagnant fluids trapped in the soft tissue.

4. **Trauma liniment** (chapter 10): Trauma liniment (die da jiu) has been used by martial artists for centuries to treat a wide variety of injuries. Trauma liniment is applied externally in combination with simple massage techniques. Alternatively, layers of gauze may be soaked in the liniment and wrapped over the injury, creating a simple poultice. Trauma liniment contains herbs that are classified as blood regulating. These herbs dispel blockages of stagnant qi and blood and prevent blood from congealing. Some herbs in this category are said to "break the blood" or to "crack stagnation," and they help to dismantle the beaver dam.

5. **Die da wan** (chapter 15): Die da wan (trauma pills), or tinctures of qi li san, can be taken internally (administered orally). These formulas are basically the internal counterparts of trauma liniment and are usually combined with ex-

Keep It Simple

At first glance, all these different choices may seem complicated, but Chinese sports medicine is basically simple and direct. Let's go back to that most common injury, the sprained ankle. When I was first learning about Chinese sports medicine, my brother sprained his ankle quite badly. It started to swell immediately. Fortunately, I had brought my first-aid kit home for the holidays. First I bled the ankle and cupped it to reduce the swelling. Three to four minutes of massage and pressure on leg acupoints like ST 36 and GB 39 (see chapter 13) further reduced the swelling. Then I applied a poultice of san huang san, which he left on overnight. I then gave him the one trauma pill that was in my kit. The next morning he was able to walk normally, with just a hint of swelling remaining.

ternal therapies in order to treat the problem from the inside and outside simultaneously.

6. **Movement and exercise:** Simple range-of-motion exercises that do not aggravate the injury are appropriate at this stage. It is vital to start these as soon as possible to prevent muscle atrophy and restore normal movement and range of motion to the injured area. Movement also helps to stimulate circulation, reducing residual swelling.

Back to the Beaver Dam

Think of each treatment modality as another way of dealing with the problem of the beaver dam.

CUPPING AND BLEEDING: Directly removes part of the dam (stagnant blood and fluids) and some of the pond backed up behind the dam. (See chapter 9 for specifics on how to use this therapy.)

SAN HUANG SAN: Helps to move the stagnant pond through the dam-reducing stagnation and inflammation. Prevents more debris (sticks, leaves, and mud) from collecting, and as stagnant fluids begin to move, cools the stagnant water behind the dam.

MASSAGE AND ACUPRESSURE: Pushes stagnant water through and around the dam.

TRAUMA LINIMENT: Aids massage in dispersing the pond but also prevents further accumulation of debris as fluid and blood begin to move.

TRAUMA PILLS: Cracks open the dam and moves stagnant fluids through.

MOVEMENT/EXERCISE: Restores the free-flowing stream to its normal path and keeps it from stagnating again.

STAGE 2—POST-ACUTE

This stage usually begins within a week after the initial injury and can last up to three weeks. The swelling and pain are reduced, and much or all of the inflammation may be gone. There is often stiffness due to spasms in tendons that have contracted reflexively in an attempt to protect the injured area by immobilizing it. In stage 1, these spasms were difficult to see and treat because of the swelling and inflammation. If the injury was treated properly in stage 1, the swelling and stiffness may be minimal at this point.

In stage 2, treatment can be more direct and aggressive. Herbal soaks and applications of wet heat that were forbidden in stage 1 can now be used. Wet heat in the form of hot towels, herbal soaks, hot tubs, or hydrocollator packs (which can be purchased at most pharmacies) penetrates muscles, tendons, and ligaments, relaxing spasms and stiffness. Herbal soaks (chapter 12) in particular can soften and disperse remaining pockets of congealed blood that can cause tissues to adhere, thereby preventing them from sliding smoothly across one another. Unless dispersed, these adhesions can limit range of motion.

Treatment

1. **Massage and acupressure:** Pressure on acupoints may be used as in stage 1, but they are accompanied by more deep direct massage techniques over the area of injury. Trauma liniment may continue to be used with massage to dispel any remaining blood stasis.

2. **Herbal soaks:** Making an herbal soak consists of cooking herbs in a pot of water and then immersing the injured area in the liquid. Soaks are very useful for wrist, ankle, hand, and foot injuries. They can be used on larger body parts by soaking towels in the liquid and applying them to the injured area. In the majority of cases, I recommend the tendon-relaxing soak (chapter 12). The herbal ingredients themselves are only slightly warming in nature, so they don't overheat the injured area. This soak also contains a

large amount of tou gu cao, an herb that helps to relax spasms in the sinews.

3. **Movement:** Restoring movement and normal function is critical at this stage. Do simple range-of-motion exercises in conjunction with exercises that strengthen and reeducate the injured area without reaggravating it. Injuries often create a break in the connection of the injured area with the rest of the body. There is a sense that the injured part is not integrated with the body as a whole. An injured knee becomes referred to as "my bad knee," as though it is other or different. The injured area must be retrained to function in harmony with the rest of the body for it to *fully* heal and re-

A Word About Tendonitis

Tendonitis is a sinew problem that develops over a period of time, usually from improper and repetitive stress on the tendons. This results in microtears at the attachments of the tendons and the bone. The tendon becomes swollen and inflamed. Rest usually relieves the pain, but each time the activity is resumed the tears are stressed again, causing more inflammation. Activity often increases the pain, but sometimes pain disappears with activity and increases when the activity stops. This is because movement and exercise bring more circulation to the local area, temporarily creating a free flow of blood and qi, which in turn reduces pain. There is usually no recollection of a specific injury and therefore no obvious acute swollen stage, although there can be chronic inflammation. Tendonitis occurs most frequently in the rotator cuff, Achilles' tendon, and elbow, although it can also occur in the knee and wrist. Carpal tunnel syndrome is a form of tendonitis in which the wrist tendon sheaths become inflamed and create pressure on the median nerve in the wrist.

By the time most people realize they have tendonitis, it is usually a chronic stage 2 or stage 3 sinew injury. Treatment consists of gentle massage at the attachment of the tendon to the bone in conjunction

duce potential for reinjury. Many of the key exercises that stimulate this reintegration, build strength, and restore range of motion are detailed in chapters 5 and 6. They can be supplemented by other exercises presented in part 4, where specific conditions are listed alphabetically by body part.

Vigorous exercise or competitive sports activities should not be resumed at this time. As pain subsides and movement is restored, the impulse to take up activities where you left off before the injury is very strong. Remember, the injured area is still weak and needs to be strengthened gradually. Slowly increase range of motion and intensity while continuing to massage the area with lini-

with warming soaks (chapter 12), plasters (chapter 11), and liniments (chapter 10). Tendon lotion, which is very warming, is often the treatment of choice, but if there is residual inflammation, less warming liniments and plasters like trauma liniment or Wu Yang pain-relieving plaster are more appropriate. So how do you know if there is still inflammation if the area is not red, hot, and swollen? If you think there is no inflammation, use a small amount of one of the warming liniments or try a warming soak. If it aggravates your tendonitis, switch to more cooling or neutral temperature herbs until the inflammation is gone.

Correct exercise is a key factor in healing tendonitis. The body must be retrained to use the muscles and tendons properly. Tendonitis is usually caused by the repetitive isolation of certain muscles, such as those involved in clicking a mouse, using a screwdriver, or hitting golf balls. Standard weight-training or resistance exercises are usually not very useful in this situation, because they also tend to be repetitive movements that isolate muscle groups. They can actually aggravate the already inflamed tendon. Gentle exercises like the Daily Dozen (chapter 5) and the Eight Brocade Plus (chapter 6), which promote circulation and reintegrate and reconnect the injured tendon with the rest of the body, are more appropriate.

ments before and after exercise. Use soaks or medicated plasters to release spasms or break up accumulations. It is often useful to stimulate ear acupoints (chapter 13) while gradually moving the injured area through range-of-motion exercises.

STAGE 3—CHRONIC

This stage begins three to four weeks after the injury. Swelling and inflammation are gone, but stiffness and aching pain may still be present. A minor sprain should be resolved by this point, especially if it was treated properly from the beginning. However, injuries to tendons and ligaments can take up to six to eight weeks to heal completely and in severe cases can take even longer. If the injury was treated properly in the acute stage, stiffness should be minimal at this point and more rigorous exercises can be initiated. This is also a time when the sinews are prone to reinjury, primarily because of the urge to try to return immediately to previous levels of

My Mother's Achilles' Tendonitis

My mother developed Achilles' Tendonitis. Various foot problems over many years probably contributed by changing the way she walked, and her calf muscles were very tight. Gradually the pain increased until she had difficulty walking. There was thickening of the tendon and calcium deposits at the attachment of the tendon to the heel. X-rays showed that a bone spur was slowly developing there. At that point she began to use the tendon-relaxing soak to ease stiffness in the tendon and soften up the calcium deposits. At night she applied 701 plasters. This warming adhesive plaster softens lumps and breaks up calcium deposits and bone spurs. She also visited a physical therapist who massaged the ankle to break up adhesions and improve circulation. He taught her stretches and exercises that helped to improve the flexibility and mobility of the ankle. Over two months the pain was gradually reduced and she was able to walk normally. This kind of multitherapy approach is critical to resolve chronic tendon problems.

performance. Runners want to return to the mileage they covered before the injury, and yoga students want to keep up with the rest of the class. Slowly increase the intensity while continuing to use the Chinese sports medicine treatments from stage 2.

After you have rested a sprain or strain for three or four weeks, it is frustrating to still feel pain and discomfort. Residual pain and stiffness and the danger of reinjury are due to several factors:

1. **There are still accumulations of qi, blood, and fluids creating stiffness and pain.** You may actually feel hard nodules like sand in the tissue, indicating accumulation and calcification. This is common in Achilles' tendonitis. Exercises that gently stretch and mobilize the tendon, soaks like the tendon-relaxing soak, and liniments and plasters that break up accumulations help to remove the remaining stasis and ease joint pain and stiffness.

2. **There may be some instability in the joint if the ligaments were overstretched, making it weak and vulnerable to reinjury.** This is very common in wrist and ankle injuries, where many small ligaments hold the bones together in a complex arrangement. These ligaments are easily sprained and overstretched, resulting in joint instability. When you rotate an unstable joint, the bones and ligaments often slip very slightly in and out of their natural alignment, creating a clicking or popping sound. Strengthening exercises are very important. The muscles around the joint must be systematically strengthened to restore stability to an area that has been structurally weakened. Tonifying herb formulas that contain herbs known to strengthen sinews and bones, such as bone-knitting powder, or patent remedies like gei jie da bu wan and tze pao san pien may also be taken to aid the body's natural repair process. These formulas are more effective if used with local application of plasters and poultices that move the blood and strengthen sinews and bones, such as the gou pi plaster or sinew-bone poultice (see chapter 11).

3. **Circulation in the injured area is impaired, and cold may have penetrated the outer layers of soft tissue.** The injury

may feel slightly cool or cold to the touch, especially when you press into it past the superficial muscle layer. The area may also feel more sensitive to the cold and ache in damp or chilly weather. In chapter 2, we saw how a chronic injury can eventually become a *bi* (obstruction) syndrome, manifesting as arthritic joint pain. Often this is the result of failure to treat the injury properly from the outset and

My Wrist Injury

I injured my wrist during a seminar taught by one of my kung fu instructors. We were practicing *chin na* (joint-locking) techniques. He had me grab him and then demonstrated a painful wrist lock. I heard a sickening crunching sound as pain shot through my wrist. I was able to go on with the class, but by the end I could hardly bend my wrist. We massaged the arm and wrapped the wrist with cloths soaked in trauma liniment. Over the next two weeks I applied gou pi plasters to move stagnation and relax the tendons and ligaments that were in spasm. My teacher then set the bones back into place. By this time the wrist felt pretty good, so I forgot about it and went back to training, but it was never quite the same. Periodically I would hear something crackle when I rotated the wrist or made a tight fist. My grip strength was weaker than it had been before. Once a year I would do something as simple as blocking a punch, there would be a crunching noise, something would slip out of place, and the wrist would lock up again. The small ligaments that bind the eight carpal (wrist) bones were overstretched each time I reinjured my wrist. Finally, after several years of merely applying first-aid treatments and not following through until the injury was completely healed, I treated my wrist properly. I used plasters that strengthen the tendons and bones while simultaneously taking bone-knitting powder. I also did the Eight Brocade Plus (chapter 6) and other exercises that helped to strengthen the wrist. When there had been no pain for weeks, I practiced some of the martial arts movements with a heavy broadsword, to further improve grip strength and joint stability.

overicing. If the injury has progressed to this stage, use warming soaks and plasters that drive out the cold and improve local circulation. Moxibustion (chapter 16) is particularly useful. Burning herbal cigars (called "moxa sticks") over acupuncture points or over cold, stiff areas helps to warm the tissues and drive out the cold. The moxa herbs themselves have blood-moving and circulation activation properties, so this therapy is more effective than heat alone. Warming liniments (chapter 10) such as tendon lotion and U-I oil are also effective when sinew injuries are aggravated by cold.

A Case of Cold Back Pain

An aikido practitioner came to my clinic with back pain. He had originally hurt his back by lifting a piece of heavy machinery, but the injury was exacerbated by aikido, a martial art that involves a great deal of throwing and rolling. On the first several visits I treated his back with massage and acupuncture, but there was little improvement. Finally I noticed that although his back felt warm to the touch on the surface, when pressed deeply, it felt cold. When I commented on this, he mentioned that the back felt more vulnerable and sensitive to cold than the rest of his body. I performed intensive moxibustion (chapter 16) on his back, heating it up until the skin started to sweat. Then I soaked paper towels in U-I oil (chapter 10) and placed them on his back. I covered the paper towels with a hydrocollator pack (a form of wet heat). One of the ingredients in U-I oil is an oil extracted from the herbs in the moxa stick. The heat from the hydrocollator pack drove the oil into the muscles. This combination turned the corner on his back pain.

Women, Menstruation, and Sinew Injuries

Premenstrual symptoms and dysmenorrhea (painful periods) are so common that most women consider them a normal part of being female. Despite the general acceptance of this point of view, in Chinese medicine these menstrual irregularities are seen as an imbalance in the movement of the qi and blood. Chinese medicine considers women to be more prone than men to imbalances involving the blood. This is due primarily to the monthly discharge of menstrual blood and the internal processes that regulate the menstrual cycle. From the standpoint of Chinese sports medicine, any imbalance in the cyclical production and discharge of blood can be a contributing factor in sinew and bone injuries and a woman's ability to heal them.

In Chinese medicine, the liver has a very important function in relation to the blood. The liver is said to store the blood. It releases blood to the sinews when the body moves from rest to activity. If the sinews are adequately supplied with blood, they are supple and flexible and can move smoothly and easily. In women, the liver also releases and helps guide blood to the uterus prior to its discharge as menstrual blood. If the liver energy is not relaxed, the normally smooth movement of qi and blood becomes blocked as it moves downward toward the uterus. This may result in bloating, breast distension, and mood swings as well as pain and cramping. Stress, overwork, emotional upset, and irregular food intake can contribute to a blockage of qi and blood on their way to the uterus. If the movement of qi and blood is impeded, there can be a relative decrease in circulation to the extremities and less nourishment supplied to the tendons. This situation can be exacerbated if the blood is inadequately replenished after the menses. This is usually the result of overtraining and a lack of nourishment from irregular or improper eating habits. The combination can lead to undernourished, dry, brittle tendons that are inadequately supplied with blood.

Menstrual irregularities that may affect the sinews and the bones can be grouped into three general categories:

QI AND BLOOD STAGNATION

- PMS symptoms such as bloating, cramping, distended and painful breasts, and mood swings.

- Pain and cramping with the menses.

- Headaches related to menstrual cycle, usually relieved by discharge of menstrual blood.

- Clots in the menstrual blood.

These symptoms indicate that the qi and blood are stagnating or blocking on the way to the uterus. Pain is the result of qi and blood not flowing smoothly and freely. Clots and severe pain may indicate the presence of stagnant blood. When the qi stagnates fluids may also stagnate, causing bloating and distension. Reducing stress and avoiding emotional upset can help the blood and qi to flow more freely. If these symptoms persist, see a practitioner of traditional Chinese medicine. Chinese medicine offers very effective treatments for pain and bloating associated with qi and blood stagnation.

PREGNANCY AND CARPAL TUNNEL SYNDROME

A significant number of women develop carpal tunnel syndrome during pregnancy. More blood and fluid is produced during pregnancy, and the fetus and amniotic fluid create a blockage (positive though it may be!) to normal circulation. As a result, it is easy for fluid to accumulate in the tissues. If fluids accumulate in the tissues of the wrist, they swell and create pressure on the median nerve in the wrist, which in turn can cause pain and numbness. This situation is worse if the arms are hanging down for long periods. Chinese medicine views this as an accumulation of qi and fluids, which occurs because of the greater demands made on the circulatory system during pregnancy. Gentle, regular exercise and massage can help the body reabsorb and circulate fluids that have accumulated in the tissues, thereby reducing pressure on the median nerve.

INSUFFICIENT BLOOD

- Cessation of period in young women or lack of menstruation.

- Periods that last only two to three days.

- Light or scanty menstrual flow.

- Fatigue after the menses.

- Anemia.

These symptoms often indicate a general deficiency of blood. The body may be failing to replenish the blood in between the menses, reducing the overall quantity of the blood. As a consequence, there is less blood to nourish the sinews. Sinews that are not nourished by the blood tend to be less pliable and more susceptible to injury. Many women who experience these symptoms are not diagnosed as anemic, yet in Chinese medicine they are still considered to be blood deficient. These symptoms can be severe, particularly in teenage girls. Health practitioners have been seeing the "female athlete triad" with increasing frequency. The triad comprises

1. insufficient caloric intake or anorexia.

2. amenorrhea (insufficient menstruation).

3. decreased bone density.

This situation is often exacerbated by overtraining, which further depletes the body's reserves. Girls who participate in sports or engage in intense physical exercise need to eat well and get plenty of rest. If they are not getting sufficient nutrients and body fat drops, they may either not develop their period or it can stop completely. Their ovaries stop producing eggs and estrogen levels drop. This can weaken bones, increasing the possibility of a stress fracture and osteoporosis later in life. Although the female triad generally occurs in younger women beginning menstruation, the general principle of this imbalance can apply to older women as well as anyone recovering from a bone fracture.

Many women with this kind of blood insufficiency are also vegetarians who have been told that eating raw foods is healthier. These women often have great difficulty healing sports injuries because their bodies cannot manufacture enough healthy blood to nourish muscles, tendons, and bones. They are starved of the nutrients that form the building blocks of blood. Often, switching to a diet that includes meat is an important part of the healing process for these women.

HEAT IN THE BLOOD AND MASSES THAT OBSTRUCT THE BLOOD

- Prolonged menstrual bleeding.

- Very heavy menstrual flow.

- Spotting between periods.

- Presence of uterine fibroids or cysts.

According to Chinese medicine, prolonged menstrual bleeding (seven days or more) and a very heavy menstrual flow can be caused by internal heat. This heat accelerates the movement of the blood, pushing it out of its channels and causing an excessive discharge of menstrual blood or breakthrough bleeding during the cycle. In Chinese medicine, uterine fibroids and cysts are often classified as congealed blood or phlegm. These hard masses can block the normal movement of the blood, causing spotting and bleeding in between the menses.

Internal heat can lead to blood deficiency if it causes a woman to lose too much blood over an extended period of time. Masses like fibroids and cysts can also cause excessive blood loss but at the same time are indicative of a stasis of energy and blood. Both scenarios can lead to reduced circulation of blood to the sinews, slowing their healing time and leaving them vulnerable to injury.

Traditional Chinese medicine can offer specific and effective treatment of the menstrual irregularities previously outlined, in contrast with the less specific hormonal therapies commonly used in Western medicine.

Often, addressing such irregularities is a key step in the healing and prevention of tendon injuries. However, because gynecological problems are complex, often involving multiple contributing factors, women should seek out experienced practitioners of Chinese medicine for treatment of these conditions.

CHAPTER 4

Down to the Bone

Fractures and How They Heal

Everyone knows that fractures are not to be trifled with. Broken bones can be serious and very painful injuries that require immediate medical attention and diagnostic tests like X-rays. Complete fractures, in which the two ends of the bone are completely separated, are extremely painful. Bones contain a rich supply of nerves and blood. This accounts for the pain and swelling that occur almost immediately after the break. Even in partial breaks such as greenstick fractures or hairline fractures, pain and swelling can be severe and persist for some time. Keep in mind that pain due to broken bones can be very different in different areas of the body and that pain thresholds vary greatly from person to person. The broken toe or rib that incapacitates one person is often shrugged off by another.

FRACTURE HEALING

Fractures are often accompanied by soft tissue (sinew) damage. The muscles, tendons, and ligaments are injured simultaneously with the bone. This is particularly true if the fracture occurs at or near a joint. It is not surprising, then, that the treatment of fractures in the acute phase is very similar to the treatment of acute sinew injuries. If you haven't read the discussion of sinew injuries in chapter 3, go back and read it now.

Chinese sports medicine divides fracture healing into three distinct stages of about two weeks each.

1. **Acute stage** (weeks one to two): During the first seven days after the bone is fractured, there is acute swelling and pain. The blood vessels around the bone also break and create a pool of blood that within a week begins to produce bone cells. By the second week, the bone has begun to knit, causing itching and discomfort that is often worse at night.

Types of Fractures

COMPLETE: The two ends of the bone are completely separated. This is sometimes referred to as "a clean break."

COMPOUND (OPEN): One end of the broken bone or a fragment of bone penetrates the skin, creating an open wound and the possibility of infection, because the bone is exposed to the outside world.

COMMINUTED: The bone is fractured into several segments of bone, some of which may be small like splinters.

AVULSION: A small particle of bone attached to a ligament or tendon is pulled away from the main surface of the bone.

COMPRESSION: A fracture caused by compressive forces squeezing or pressing on the bone in both directions. This is most commonly seen in spinal vertebrae.

SPIRAL: A curved, twisting, or shearing of the bone. This is common in skiing and in-line skating, where a fall can create a twisting force that fractures the leg where it is held by the boot.

2. **Knitting stage** (weeks three to four): This is a continuation of the end of the acute phase. The bones continue to knit as more and more bone cells are formed. By the fourth week, the bones may have knit but are still soft and flexible at the site of the break.

3. **Complete healing** (weeks five to six): In a simple complete ("clean") break, if the individual is healthy, the bones should be solid and strong by the end of the sixth week. More severe breaks may take longer, but correct treatment from the outset can greatly speed the healing process.

GREENSTICK: A type of partial fracture that usually occurs in children, whose bones are still flexible and bend before they break. Greenstick fractures are named for their resemblance to a live twig that is bent. The break occurs on the far side of the bend and does not go all the way through the bone. These fractures heal relatively quickly.

HAIRLINE CRACK: A slight crack on the surface of the bone. A hairline crack is a partial fracture that is difficult to detect with X-rays. Although it is usually considered minor, I know of one kickboxer whose femur was cracked by a kick. Marrow leaked from the crack onto the nerves in the leg, a very serious injury requiring surgery.

STRESS FRACTURE: A hairline crack in the bone caused by overtraining or repetitive stress. These fractures usually occur in the lower leg or the foot. They are very common in runners. Stress fractures were originally called "marching fractures" because they frequently occurred in soldiers who marched long distances with heavy packs. Often with stress fractures there is no visible swelling or lump to indicate the presence of a fracture.

TREATMENT

Acute Stage

Treatment in the acute stage is much like the treatment of sinew injuries in chapter 3. The main focus of treatment at this point is to reduce swelling and inflammation while promoting free flow of qi and blood. San huang san combined with trauma pills is the treatment of choice. Gentle massage above and below the site of the break is also very helpful in reducing swelling and restoring the free flow of circulation. If the break is severe, only light stroking movements may be tolerable. Pressure on acupressure points and ear points (chapter 13) can be used to kill pain and stimulate the body's healing response. If a rib is fractured, the rib fracture formula (chapter 15) is used along with plasters like yunnan paiyao plaster (chapter 11). Self-adhering medicated plasters generally work well on areas like the ribs where poultices and wraps can be messy and hard to apply.

Soft Casts Speed Up Healing

In China there is a long tradition of using soft casts or splints to immobilize broken bones. This was not because of primitive conditions, but because soft casts and splints have certain inherent advantages. Chinese bonesetters often employed a complex form of splinting that allowed varying amounts of pressure to be applied to different parts of the bone, thereby encouraging a crooked bone to knit straight. This could be done even two to three weeks after the break when the knitting bones were still soft. Although soft casts are used more frequently today, doctors are sometimes reluctant to use them because of the possibility of rebreaking the bone when it is only partially knit. However, if you are careful, a soft removable cast will allow you to apply the herbal liniments and poultices used in Chinese sports medicine directly over the break. A soft cast also allows you to receive massage and acupuncture and to begin rehabilitative exercise sooner.

Trauma liniment (chapter 10) can be used as a substitute for san huang san. Although it cannot be massaged directly over the site of a fresh fracture, it can be applied by soaking gauze or clean cloth in the liniment and applying it as a poultice. *Trauma liniment and other liniments, poultices, and plasters cannot be used in a compound fracture, where the bone has penetrated the skin, creating an open wound, or over any skin lacerations that may accompany a fracture.*

Exercise generally begins as soon as swelling and pain have subsided. Until the end of the acute phase, exercise consists primarily of isometric muscle contractions. Larger, stronger movements cannot be attempted until the bone is more fully knit.

Knitting Stage

In a healthy individual who gets plenty of rest and proper nutrition, the bones will knit on their own, particularly if they were treated properly in the acute stage. During the knitting stage, there are three primary goals in treatment:

Atrophy

Muscle atrophy is one of the major causes of reinjury and residual complaints after an injury. Atrophy actually begins within three to four days of disuse. That is why it is vital to reduce swelling as soon as possible and begin rehabilitative exercises as soon as the swelling stops. Weakened muscles cause the body to compensate. This can cause injuries in other parts of the body. It is not uncommon for an athlete with an ankle injury to develop knee or hip pain in the opposite leg from subtly shifting weight away from the injury. A friend of mine fractured his patella. There was no soft tissue damage and the injury healed perfectly, but six weeks in a cast caused tremendous atrophy in the leg. Because he did not follow through with a progressive strengthening program, he injured his ankle and the soft tissue of the knee when he returned to sports too soon.

1. Encourage the bones to mend.

2. Remove any residual stasis and promote local circulation.

3. Minimize muscle atrophy.

Bone-knitting powder (chapter 15) is the key herbal formula in the knitting stage. Formulas like this have been used for centuries by the Shaolin monks to speed bone healing and to mend fractures that were healing slowly. I have used this formula with hundreds of people, many of whom had fractures that failed to heal, either because the body's resources were too weak or because the damage was too extensive. I saw one elderly woman with a fracture that had still not healed after eight weeks in a cast. She took bone-knitting powder for three weeks and was able to get rid of the cast and resume her normal activities. Bone-knitting powder contains many herbs that work synergistically to

The Nine Herbs That Help Heal Broken Bones

These herbs are never taken individually to treat broken bones. They are usually part of a comprehensive formula like bone-knitting powder that harmonizes the blood and tonifies the kidneys and the liver in order to strengthen the bones.

1. GU SUI BU (literally "mender of shattered bone"): *Rhizoma gusuibu;* drynaria. *Action:* Tonifies the kidneys and strengthens sinew and bones.

2. BU GU ZHI (literally "tonify bone resin"): *Fructus psoraleae corylifoliae;* scuffy pea. *Action:* Tonifies the kidneys and strengthens sinew and bones.

3. XU DUAN (literally "restore the broken"): *Radix dipsaci;* Japanese teasel root. *Action:* Tonifies the kidneys and strengthens sinew and bones.

- tonify the qi and blood so that the bones are properly nourished and supplied with necessary nutrients.

- remove blood stasis and promote circulation.

- tonify the kidneys, which in turn strengthen and heal the broken bone. This is due to the energetic connection between the kidneys and the bones. Bone-knitting powder contains six of the nine herbs known for centuries to help the body heal broken bones.

In sinew injuries, herbal soaks are very important to relax sinews and break up accumulations of congealed blood. However, with fractures, soaks can actually be detrimental. Many of the blood-dispersing, spasm-relaxing soaks mentioned in chapters 3 and 12 can actually prevent bones from healing because they have a dispersing, spreading effect on the qi and blood, whereas herbal

4. DU ZHONG: *Cortex eucommiae ulmoidis;* eucommia bark. *Action:* Tonifies the kidneys and strengthens sinew and bones.

5. GOU JI: *Rhizoma cibotii barometz;* cibotium. *Action:* Tonifies the kidneys, disperses cold, and strengthens sinew and bones.

6. GUI BAN: *Plastrum testudinis;* land tortoise shell. *Action:* Tonifies the kidneys and strengthens the bone matrix.

7. HE GU: *Os tigris;* tiger bone. (As tigers are an endangered species, dog or cat bone is usually substituted.) *Action:* Disperses cold and damp. Strengthens sinew and bones. Useful for arthralgic pain that is worse with cold and damp weather.

8. TU BIE CHONG: *Eupolyphagae seu opisthoplatiae;* wingless cockroach. *Action:* Breaks up congealed blood. Particularly useful in cases of fracture or sinew injury.

9. ZI RAN TONG (literally "natural copper"): pyrite. *Action:* Disperses congealed blood and promotes healing of sinews and bones.

formulas that help heal broken bones have a consolidating action that concentrates the qi and blood. During the knitting stage, stagnant blood must still be cleared from the injured area. Herbs like zi ran tong and tu bie chong, which break up stagnation but do not interfere with the knitting process, are used for this purpose.

Massage and exercise are extremely important therapies in the knitting stage, as they promote circulation and prevent atrophy of muscle tissue. Massage can be performed above and below the break. Exercises at this stage include isometric muscle contraction as well as range-of-motion and strength-building exercises in the surrounding joints. For example, in the case of a fractured patella (kneecap), tensing the thigh muscles exercises the hamstrings and the quadriceps, while range-of-motion exercises and strength training for the hip and ankle will keep muscles in these areas from atrophying. If possible, do some gentle aerobic exercise like walking (if the fracture is in the upper body) or exercises that build internal strength like the Eight Brocade Plus (chapter 6). If the fracture is in the lower body, the Eight Brocade Plus can be done seated. Walking and internal exercises help to circulate the qi and blood. This can speed healing and prevent stasis.

Moxibustion (chapter 16) is a warming therapy that helps to drive out cold and dampness that can easily penetrate damaged tissue. It also stimulates circulation and can help to move static blood and qi. It is useful toward the end of the knitting stage, when swelling and inflammation are gone.

Look out for infection! A not uncommon culprit in a fracture that does not heal is an infection in the bone. Infections are more likely to occur in compound fractures where the bone has penetrated the skin, exposing it to the open air. They are also more likely to occur in diabetics or where there is a preexisting circulation problem or chronic edema. If the injured area remains red, puffy, and painful after several weeks, see your doctor as soon as possible.

Complete Healing Stage

By week five, the bones should be knit but are still hardening and consolidating. At this stage tonic herbs that tonify the kidneys and the qi and blood can help the healing and prevent arthritic pains later in life. In children, these kinds of formulas are usually unnecessary, because a healthy child gets plenty of rest and has more than enough excess energy to divert a sufficient amount of the body's resources to heal the break. Adults, on the other hand, who are stressed, overworked, not eating well, and not getting enough sleep may not have the extra energy needed to heal properly. As a result, the healing process is slowed. Tonic formulas can be very useful in these instances.

Usually these kinds of herbal formulas need to be administered by a qualified practitioner of traditional Chinese medicine who matches the formula to an individual's constitution. This is particularly true for children. If it is not possible to see an herbalist, there are two tonic formulas that I have found to be extremely effective in fractures that are slow to heal. Gei jie da bu wan and tze pao san pien are both broad-spectrum tonics that strongly supplement the body's energy during the healing process. These pills *should not* be administered to children. In a healthy adult who is not on any medication, they can be taken safely for a two-to-three-week period to help the bones knit completely. They *should not* be taken for extended periods unless prescribed by a qualified practitioner of traditional Chinese medicine. One of my students had a hairline fracture of the sternum from a flying side kick to the chest. This is a difficult injury to heal. Although he received acupuncture and he rested, at the end of six weeks there was still residual pain and soreness that did not seem to be diminishing. Ten days of tze pao san pien pills allowed him to return to training.

PART II

Injury Prevention:

Exercise, Diet, and Health Preservation

INTRODUCTION TO PART II

The ancient Chinese observed that those born with a weak constitution could become strong and vital through proper exercise and
diet and the adoption of a lifestyle that conserved, rather than depleted, the body's resources. They also observed that those born
with a strong constitution could become weak and ill if these same
principles were not followed.

In one of the oldest books on Chinese medicine, the *Huang Ti
Nei Jing*, Emperor Huang-ti asks his adviser why the people of
today are not as vital and do not live as long as the people of ancient times. His adviser's answer outlines the basic principles of
healthy living, diet, and exercise that even today form one of the
cornerstones of traditional Chinese medicine. Working from these
concepts, many generations of doctors developed unique methods
of exercise and conducted extensive research on the effects of diet
and food on human health. These studies led some of China's
most famous physicians to conclude that the highest forms of
medicine are those that preempt disease before it can occur. Therefore a balanced diet, exercise, and a harmonious balanced lifestyle
came to be considered superior to other forms of therapy that treat
disease only after it has already taken root in the body.

This idea, that the promotion of health, rather than the treatment of disease, is the preeminent function of medicine, led China
to embrace a different model of health from that which developed
in the West. In China, healthy elderly people who were fit and
strong into old age are held up as the standard of health, and their

exercise regimes and living habits are extolled as the secrets of longevity. Martial arts practitioners adopted many of these health secrets and incorporated them into their training programs, because they proved not only to prolong life, but to prevent injuries, speed healing, and develop a supple body capable of powerful movements. This knowledge gradually became part of Chinese sports medicine as we know it today.

Participation in sports and even the performance of many daily activities require a certain degree of physical fitness. Physical fitness is not just a function of jogging or the performance of calisthenics. It is the development of a strong, supple body that is adequately rested with reserves of energy and fueled by nourishing foods. A body that has these characteristics can perform at maximum efficiency with less chance of injury. In this section of the book, you will discover the keys to developing flexibility and strength and to maintaining maximum health through proper diet and healthy living.

CHAPTER 5

Stretching and Flexibility

When we think of flexibility, we tend to imagine a gymnast stretching in a full split or yoga practitioners who bend their bodies like pretzels. By implication, flexibility is something out of reach of the ordinary person. Outside of sports or yoga, many people rarely think of stretching except as something to do briefly after getting out of bed in the morning or following a long plane flight. Meanwhile, sports and exercise enthusiasts promote hundreds of different stretching routines, and health journals continue to debate the pros and cons of stretching before exercise. As a result, many people are confused about stretching. Should they stretch? How much? Is it better to stretch before or after exercising?

THE PROBLEM WITH STRETCHING

Part of the confusion about stretching is the word itself. "Stretching" conveys the idea of grasping the ends of a rope or a rubber band and pulling it taut. If you do this to a muscle, you can actually cause the muscle to contract rather than stretch or, worse yet, tear muscle fibers. In more than twenty years as a martial arts instructor, I have seen countless students attempt to increase flexibility through forced stretching exercises, like the classic "hurdler's stretch." Often there is little or no improvement in general flexibility, and not infrequently microscopic tears are created in the muscles, causing them to contract. More than one study has indicated that many people who stretch in order to prevent injury actually injure themselves while stretching.

Like the athletes of today, martial arts practitioners in ancient times recognized the need for exercises that improve and maintain flexibility. By observing natural phenomena, they made simple but profound observations. One of these observations was that movement kept the body's functions from stagnating. There is a famous saying in China that expresses this concept: "The hinge of the door that is opened and closed every day will never rust." A good example of this idea is frozen shoulder, a condition in which a person loses the ability to lift his or her arm overhead. The Chinese call frozen shoulder "fifty-year-old shoulder" because it often occurs in people in their fifties who simply stop raising their arm overhead. Either they injure their arm and, to protect it, restrict the range of motion, or their daily life activities don't require overhead movements. The less they move the arm, the less they are able to move it.

To prevent the kind of stagnation and inflexibility that occurs in frozen shoulder, exercises were developed by observing and imi-

The Stretch Reflex

Our muscles are not rubber bands or ropes that can be stretched out by pulling on the ends. In fact, muscles and tendons have a self-protective mechanism that works to prevent a sudden or forced stretch of the muscle tissue from occurring. Muscle spindles connect to muscle cells. When muscle cells stretch, the muscle spindles stretch with them. If the muscle stretches to the point where its integrity is endangered, the muscle spindle sends a signal to the muscle cell to contract. This is known as the "stretch reflex." The stretch reflex permits voluntary stretches that are not too sudden or forced. The tendons have similar protective mechanisms that prevent the tendons from being damaged through overstretching.

tating animals that were admired for their ease of movement. The Chinese recognized that although we cannot move exactly like animals, the essence of their movements could be captured and adapted to the human form. The deer was celebrated for its delicate steps and nimble leaps, the snake for its pliability, the monkey for its playful agility, and the tiger for its power, strength, and courage.

Like many people who like cats, I have always been fascinated by the way cats move. They appear to be lazy and sleep a lot, yet they are agile, flexible, and strong. Cats don't do stretching exercises or engage in weight training, yet they move with a supple, relaxed grace that few humans can match. Suppleness is in many ways a more useful term than flexibility or stretching. The word *supple* conjures up an image of a body that is like a piece of pliable cloth or leather, able to bend or move in any direction without kinking or binding. What the Chinese saw in the cat's movement was that cats subtly and efficiently exercise their whole body even in their simplest movements. They are supple not because they do stretching exercises, but because they relax the muscles that are unnecessary to perform a particular movement. Relaxing these "antagonistic" muscles not only allows a joint or a limb greater freedom of movement, it also creates more efficient movement that conserves the body's energy.

Agonist: The muscle that is directly engaged in the contraction, as distinguished from the *antagonistic* muscles, which have to relax at the same time for the contraction to occur. For example, when you bend your elbow the bicep muscles are the agonists, while the triceps, which must relax for the biceps to contract, are the antagonists.

The Greek root of this word is *agon,* meaning "contest" or "struggle." It is interesting that even in our language we view the movement of our muscles as a contest or tug-of-war rather than a unified harmonious action.

MIND AND MOVEMENT

The natural movement of animals and the realization that flexibility could be increased by relaxing the antagonistic muscles, rather than by stretching, were only part of what the Chinese observed. It was not only what the animals did externally that made them supple and pliable, but what they did internally. When the cat moves it is fully involved in what it is doing. Cats do not exercise while thinking about something else or watch television while running on a treadmill. Martial arts masters express this fully engaged attentiveness as being "like a cat catching a rat." When a cat stalks a rat or a mouse, it crouches with the spirit of its whole being focused on the task at hand. Mental involvement in the movements being performed engages the whole being in the exercise, producing far greater results than merely performing them by rote.

BREATHING AND FLEXIBILITY

The last and perhaps most powerful and profound thing that the Chinese observed was that animals breathe when they move. This seems absurdly obvious, but go to the gym and see how many people forget to breathe while stretching or lifting a heavy weight. We tend to take breathing for granted most of the time, yet it exerts a powerful influence on us with each inhalation and exhalation.

The snake is the master breather of the animal world. In China, the snake is celebrated for its suppleness and pliability. A snake's very movement is such a seamless blend of contraction and relaxation that it appears to flow across the ground. When snakes breathe, they breathe with their whole body, indicating that the qi moves smoothly and unimpeded in every part of their body.

Deep, relaxed diaphragmatic breathing is like the breathing of the snake. With practice it can be felt in every part of the body. This kind of breathing actually helps relax tight muscles and can increase the range of motion in joints by allowing the qi and blood to flow freely. Besides aiding flexibility, breathing into the lower abdomen helps connect the strength of the lower limbs and back to the actions of the upper arms. This brings together the overall power of the human body into a single unified action. It comes as no surprise, therefore, that breathing exercises have been a part of martial arts training for centuries.

Many people have forgotten how to breathe with their whole body. Rather than letting the diaphragm drop and the belly expand outward on inhalation, they breathe into their chest. This creates tension in the upper back, neck, and shoulders. The scalene muscles of the neck actually connect to the tops of the lungs (the plural dome). When we breathe shallowly, they are called upon to contract to help lift the top of the lung. Over time they become chronically tight. Tight neck muscles are very common in people with asthma as wheezing forces them to engage the neck muscles

The Power of the Breath

From a structural standpoint alone, the act of breathing is felt throughout the entire body. In inhalation, the intercostal muscles between the ribs contract and lift the ribs, enlarging the diameter of the thorax. This allows the diaphragm to drop and flatten, increasing the depth of the chest and creating space for air to fill the lungs. In exhalation, the intercostal muscles relax, allowing the diaphragm to spring up and push air out of the lungs.

The diaphragm arises from the lumbar vertebrae, the lower ribs, and the sternum. It arches upward into the chest like a dome. Many of the organs of digestion connect to the diaphragm. The esophagus passes through the diaphragm to connect to the stomach. The liver, stomach, and colon all have soft tissue connections with the diaphragm and are affected by its pistonlike movement. There is evidence that diaphragmatic breathing (in which the lower abdomen puffs out on inhalation) actually helps peristalsis and digestion and aids venous return of blood to the heart.

On a cellular level, the heart and lungs oxygenate the blood and dispel the waste products of cellular metabolism. Oxygen brought to the cells by the blood is the key that unlocks ATP (adenosine triphosphate), the stored energy of the cells and the biochemical activator of muscle contraction.

to help them breathe. Try a simple experiment. Breathe shallowly in a panting movement for thirty seconds. Feel how tension begins to build in your upper body. Then try breathing naturally and deeply, letting the lower abdomen relax outward with the inhalation. Feel how the body relaxes and the neck and shoulder tension starts to let go. Many athletes I have worked with found that diaphragmatic breathing increased their athletic performance across the board. A karate practitioner told me he got out of breath quickly with intensive exercise. If he biked up a steep hill, he would feel very winded, and even after he stopped it would take a long time for his breathing to return to normal. I noticed he seemed to breathe only in his chest and showed him how to breathe naturally in the diaphragm. Within several months of just adding diaphragmatic breathing to his routine, he found he did not get out of breath. He could bike up the same hills and not be

Breathing and Back Pain

Natural diaphragmatic breathing (hereafter referred to as "natural breathing") is an indispensable part of restoring injured areas to normal function. When your back "goes out," even small movements can be excruciatingly painful. You want to hold the body stiffly and breathe shallowly to avoid moving the injured area. However, because the diaphragm has connective tissue attachments to the lumbar spine, breathing can actually help restore normal movement.

One patient who came to our clinic had several herniated discs and her back hurt constantly, even at night when lying flat. Her sleep was regularly interrupted by the pain. She had long ago stopped breathing deeply into the back and lower abdomen because any attempt to do so created movement and pain in the injured area. I encouraged her to do breathing exercises. The first breaths were painful, yet she persisted, and despite the discomfort, the muscles in her back began to relax. Daily practice of breathing exercises helped restore movement to her lower back so that she could engage in more rigorous physical activity.

at all out of breath. When his doctor gave him a lung capacity test, he scored higher than anyone they had tested in years.

The lessons of the animals—natural relaxed movement, mental attention, and breathing—gradually became codified into groups of exercises that could serve as a set of warm-up exercises and simultaneously teach the body to operate more efficiently. Martial arts teachers employ these exercise routines to develop flexibility and to reeducate the body's most basic movements so that they become connected, supple, and natural. In this regard, the exercises act as a kind of neuromuscular reprogramming of our most primal movements.

The exercises that follow, which I call "the Daily Dozen," appear to be a simple set of warming-up exercises that can be done in fifteen to twenty minutes, yet if performed properly, they can help us to develop some of the pliability and grace of the lazy cat.

THE DAILY DOZEN

The Basics

There are a few basic things to remember when performing the Daily Dozen:

- The *stance* is natural, with the feet about shoulder width apart and the knees slightly bent unless otherwise specified.

- The *head* is erect, as though suspended by a thread from the top of the head.

- The *tailbone* drops under, as though attached to a plumb line. This allows a slight bending to occur at the hip joints.

- The *shoulders* relax and drop.

- The *tongue tip* is on the roof of the mouth.

- *Breathe* through the nose, using natural diaphragmatic breathing. Do not force the breath.

- Relax the *chest*.

- The *mind* is fully engaged in the movements, watching and listening to the body.

- *Movements* are slow and relaxed, without any excess tension.

- *Repetitions.* There is no fixed number of repetitions for each exercise. The numbers given here are merely general guidelines. More is not necessarily better.

Preparation

Each time you practice, put a hand on your lower abdomen and breathe naturally for several breaths, letting the mind and body calm down and relax. Feel the lower abdomen push out against your hand with each inhalation. Do not force the breath. Just let the lungs empty and fill and observe what happens. Feel as though the whole body is breathing.

1: Neck

Part I—Neck Rotation
Start: Stand facing forward with the heels together and the arms at your sides.

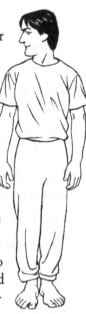

1. Slowly turn your head to the right as you inhale. Keep the neck muscles as relaxed as possible, so that you are not forcing the head to turn but *letting* it turn. Picture the spine as you use the breath to help the muscles of the torso relax. Try to feel as though a rod runs from the tip of the tailbone to the top of the head. When you turn your head, the whole spine turns on this axis. (Figure 2.)

2. Exhale and slowly turn your head back to face front. Keep the neck and torso relaxed and feel the whole spine turning as you return to the start position. (Figure 3.)

Figure 2.

3. Repeat, turning to the left side. Continue performing 4–6 repetitions on each side.

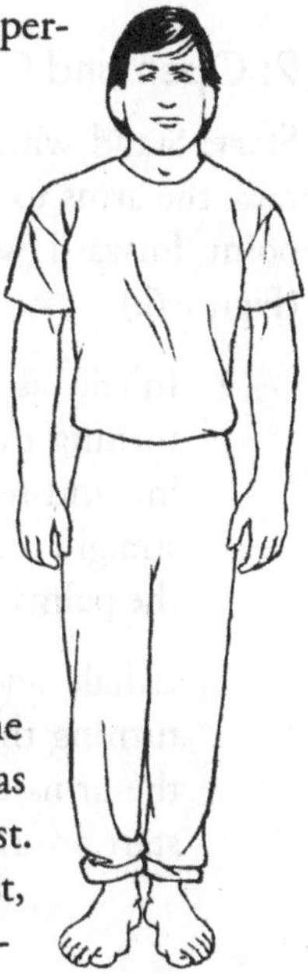

Part II—Neck Flexion and Extension

1. Inhale as you slowly raise the chin toward the ceiling. Extend the top of the head upward and backward so that the neck is lengthened. As you raise your chin, relax the front of the neck and the torso. Feel a gentle stretch running down the body to the pubic bone. (Figure 4.)

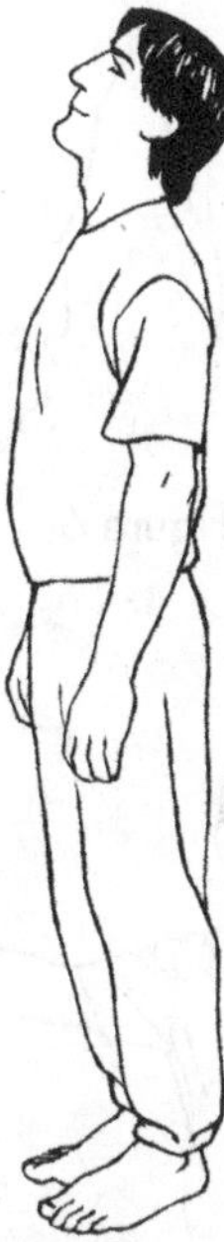

2. Exhale and bring the top of the head forward and downward as the chin moves toward the chest. Do not force the chin to the chest, just move it in that general direction as you lengthen the neck through the top of the head. Picture that you are pointing the depression at the base of the skull toward the ceiling. As you do this, relax the back of the neck and the torso and feel a gentle stretch running down the body to the tailbone. (Figure 5.)

Figure 3.

3. Repeat 4–6 times and end in the start position.

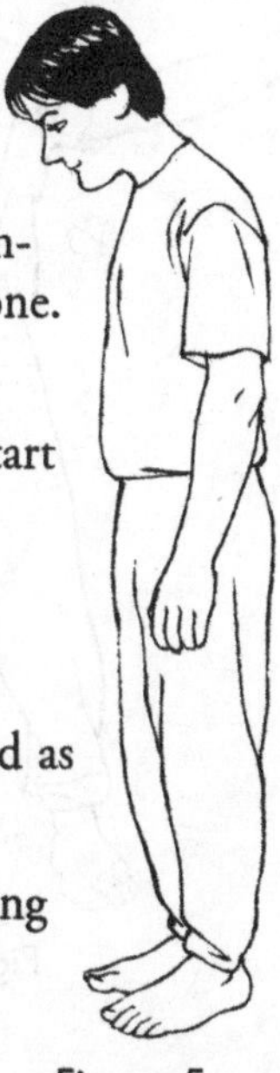

Figure 4.

Important Points

• Make sure the muscles of the neck are as relaxed as possible.

• Let the head and neck turn rather than forcing them to turn.

Figure 5.

2: Open and Close

Start: Stand with the feet shoulder width apart and raise the arms to shoulder height so that the fingers point forward with the palms facing downward. (Figure 6.)

1. Inhale as you move the arms apart, slowly turning them palms upward. Continue inhaling and separating the arms until they point straight outward to the sides of the body with the palms facing up. (Figures 7 and 8.)

2. Exhale and reverse the movement, slowly turning the palms downward as you move the arms toward each other. Finish in the start position. (Figure 6.)

    3. Repeat 8–10 times.

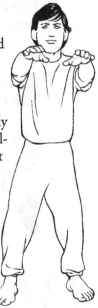

Figure 6.

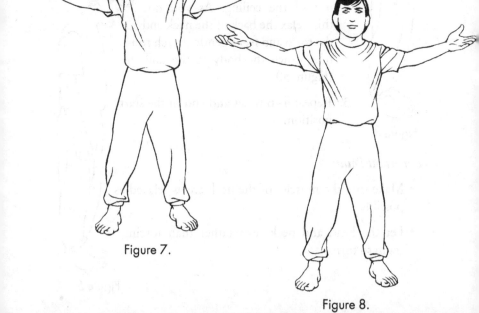

Figure 7.

Figure 8.

Important Points

- Keep the shoulders relaxed

- In the opening movement feel as though you initiate the movement from the center of the back, and in the closing movement feel as though you initiate the movement from the center of the chest.

- Coordinate the breathing with the movement. For example, as you begin to inhale, start to separate the arms. As you finish inhaling, the arms finish their outward movement.

3: Arm Rotation

Start: Stand with feet shoulder width apart, facing forward, arms at your sides.

1. Make a loose fist with the left hand and slowly raise it to the front as you inhale. (Figure 9.)

2. Continue inhaling as you lift the arm overhead. (Figure 10.) Exhale as the arm extends to the rear and back to the starting point, completing a 360-degree circle. (Figures 11 and 12.)

3. After 6–10 repetitions, reverse the direction of the circle, performing 6–10 repetitions. Remember to inhale as the arm is rising upward and exhale as the arm lowers back to the start point.

4. Repeat with the right arm.

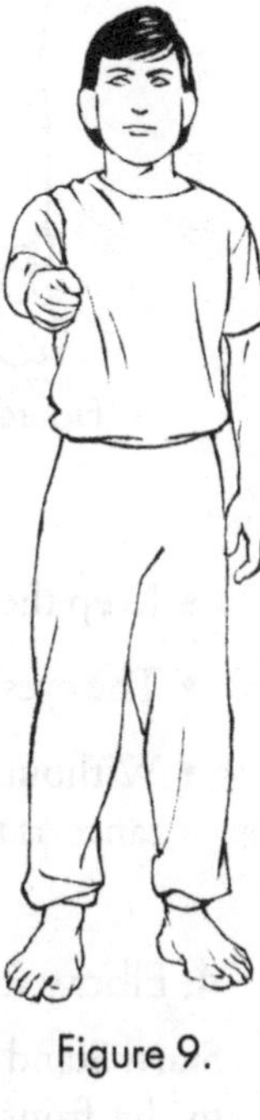

Figure 9.

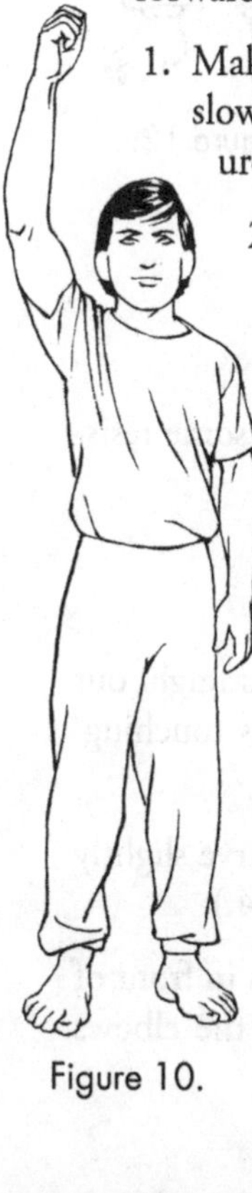

Important Points

- Keep the elbows relaxed and slightly bent.

Figure 10.

- Try not to raise the shoulders when raising the arm.

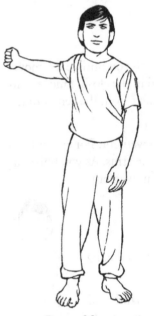

Figure 11.

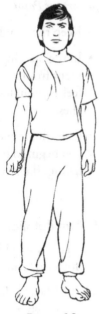

Figure 12.

- Keep the neck muscles relaxed.

- The eyes look straight ahead throughout the exercise.

- Without using muscular tension, imagine there is some resistance as though the arms are moving through water.

4: Elbow Rotation

Start: Stand with your heels together. Extend the arms straight out to the front. The palms face upward with the pinkies touching. The elbows are relaxed and slightly bent. (Figure 13.)

1. Inhale and let the elbows bend as the hands curve slightly upward and inward toward your chin. (Figure 14.)

2. As the hands pass your chin and drop, they pass in front of the chest. The backs of the hands touch and the elbows swing outward. (Figure 15.)

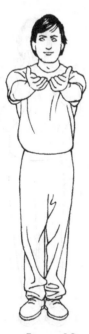

Figure 13.

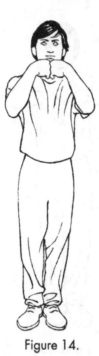

Figure 14.

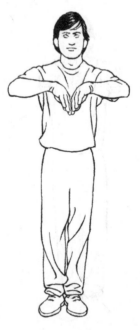

Figure 15.

3. Begin to exhale as the arms start to extend and slightly rise, palms turning to face downward. At this point, the thumb and index fingers of the two hands connect with each other. (Figure 16.)

4. Continue exhaling as the arms complete their extension, letting the shoulders get pulled forward by the motion so that the weight of the body comes forward toward the balls of the feet. (Figure 17.)

5. Begin to inhale as the hands turn palm up with the pinkies touching. (Figure 13.)

6. Repeat 6–10 times.

7. Reverse the movements. Inhale and curve the hands inward and downward toward the chest. The

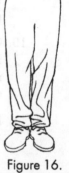

Figure 16.

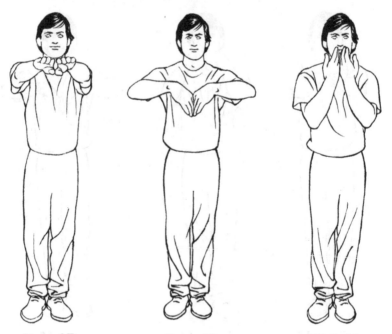

Figure 17.   Figure 18.   Figure 19.

backs of the hands touch and the elbows swing outward. (Figure 18.)

8. Finish inhaling as the hands pass the chin and the pinkies come together. (Figure 19.)

9. Exhale and begin to extend the arms outward and slightly downward, palms rotating so that the thumbs and index fingers of the two hands connect with each other and the palms face downward. (Figure 20.)

10. Continue exhaling as the arms complete their extension and let the shoulders get pulled forward by the motion so that weight of the body comes forward toward the balls of the feet. (Figure 21.)

11. Repeat 6–10 times.

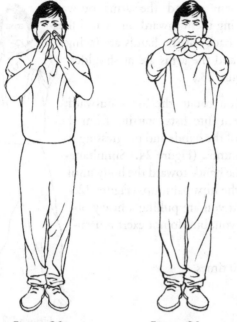

Figure 20.   Figure 21.

Important Points

- Feel how as the arms extend, the shoulders rotate, engaging the muscles of the back.

- Let this motion pull you forward toward the balls of your feet.

- Keep the elbow and shoulder joints soft and relaxed.

5: Pulling Nine Oxen

Start: Stand with the feet about shoulder width apart. The hands are in fists palm up at your lower ribs. (Figure 22.)

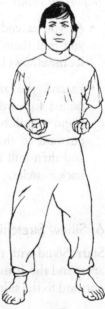

Figure 22.

1. Exhale as you extend the arms outward, slowly rotating them inward, until at full extension the backs of the hands are facing each other and the arms are at shoulder height. (Figure 23.)

2. Inhale as you rotate the arms outward, drawing them into fists, starting from the pinkie side of the hands and progressing toward the thumbs. (Figure 24.) Simultaneously pull the hands toward the body until they reach the hips palm up. (Figure 22.) Imagine that you are pulling a heavy object toward you, but do not exert muscular tension.

3. Repeat 8–10 times.

Important Points

• As you extend the arms outward and as you pull them back to the start position, let the elbows brush along the ribs.

• Extend the arms until the shoulders are pulled forward and rotate inward. As you begin to pull backward, rotate the shoulders outward so that the elbows face downward and then pull toward you, using the torso and back muscles.

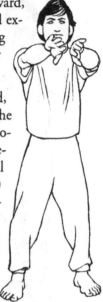

Figure 23.

6: Sinew Stretching

Start: Stand with the feet about shoulder width apart and the arms at shoulder height extended outward to the sides, palms facing downward.

1. Extend through the fingers of the right hand as though you were being pulled by your fingertips. Let the ribs extend

Figure 24.

toward the right.
As you turn the
right palm up-
ward, the left palm
turns to face backward.
(Figure 25.) Feel as though your
arms are a taut rope that is being
pulled and twisted from one end. The
pull extends from the fingertips of the
right hand through the shoulders
and ribs and down to the fingertips
of the left hand.

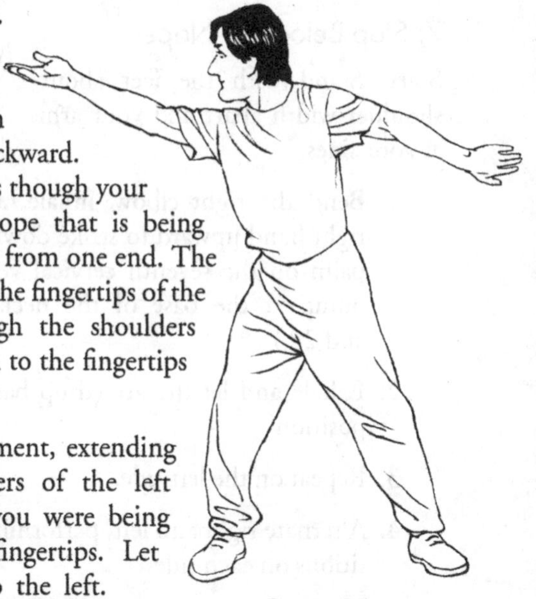

2. Reverse the movement, extending
   through the fingers of the left
   hand as though you were being
   pulled by your fingertips. Let
   the ribs extend to the left.
   As you turn the left palm
   to face upward,

Figure 25.

the right palm faces backward. (Figure 26.)

3. Repeat 6–8 times on
   each side, alternating
   sides.

Important Points

- Keep the shoulders, chest, and ribs relaxed.

  - Feel as though the body is being pulled and
    twisted like a rope rather than that you are
    forcing the joints and muscles to perform the
    action.

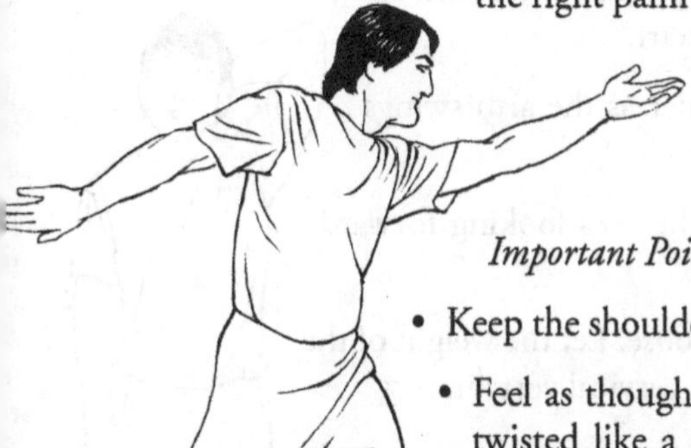

Figure 26.

7: Slap Below the Nape

Start: Stand with the feet about shoulder width apart and your arms at your sides.

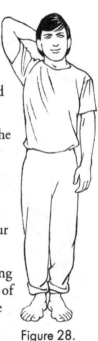

1. Bend the right elbow, inhale, and swing the right hand upward to strike downward with the palm on the seventh cervical vertebra (the big bump at the base of the neck). (Figures 27 and 28.)

2. Exhale and let the arm drop back to the start position.

3. Repeat on the left side.

4. Alternate right and left, performing 15–20 repetitions on each side.

Important Points

Figure 27.

- Inhale as the arm swings upward to slap and exhale as the arm returns to start.

- Try not to raise the shoulder as the arm swings upward.

- Keep the head erect and the eyes looking forward throughout the exercise.

- Keep the arm relaxed and loose. Let the weight of the arm fall to slap the seventh cervical vertebra.

8: Body Slapping

Start: Stand with the feet shoulder width apart and your arms at your sides.

1. Rotate the waist to the left, letting the arms swing so that the palm of the right hand slaps the top of the trapezius muscle of the left shoulder while

Figure 28.

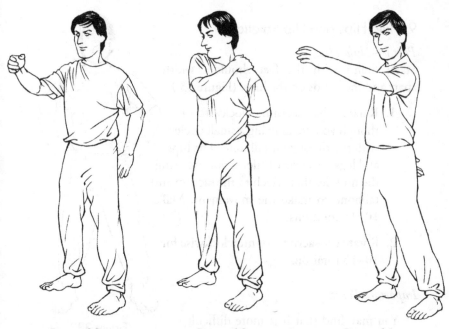

Figure 29.   Figure 30.   Figure 31.

the back of the left hand strikes the bottom of
the right shoulder blade. (Figures 29 and 30.)

2. Immediately let the waist rotate to the right so
   that the palm of the left hand strikes the top of
   the trapezius muscle of the right shoulder
   while the back of the right hand strikes the
   bottom of the left shoulder blade. (Figures 31
   and 32.)

Important Points

- Let the arms swing like ropes driven by the turning of the waist.

- The hands should strike their respective points at
  the same moment.

- The breathing is not coordinated in any particular way with the movements.

Figure 32.

9: Hula Hips and Hip Rotation

Part I—Hula Hips

Start: Stand with the feet shoulder width apart and the hands on the hips. (Figure 33.)

1. Rotate the sacrum clockwise as though you are drawing a small circle with the tip of your tailbone. The hips and legs move very little, as you are using the muscles that attach to the sacrum and tailbone to make the movement. Make 10–15 rotations.

2. Rotate the sacrum counterclockwise for 10–15 rotations.

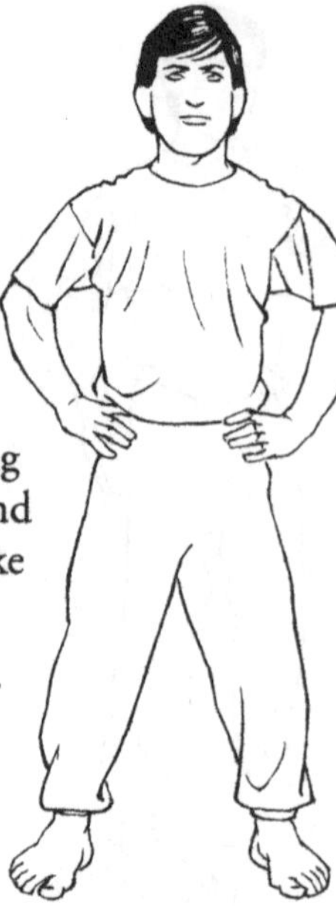

Important Points

Figure 33.

- You may find that it is more difficult to achieve a smooth rotation in one part of the circle or in one direction. Relax and let the tailbone sink downward, making as complete a circle as possible without tensing and without using muscular tension to force the movement.

- Breathe naturally.

Part II—Hip Rotation

Start: Stand with the feet shoulder width apart, palms on the sides of the waist with the thumbs facing forward and resting on the top of the hip and the middle fingers meeting on the center of the spine. (Figure 34.)

1. Turn the waist clockwise in a circle, going to the right, the front, the left, and the rear, keeping the head relatively still. (Figures 35–38.) Repeat 8–10 times.

2. Turn the waist in the opposite direction 8–10 times.

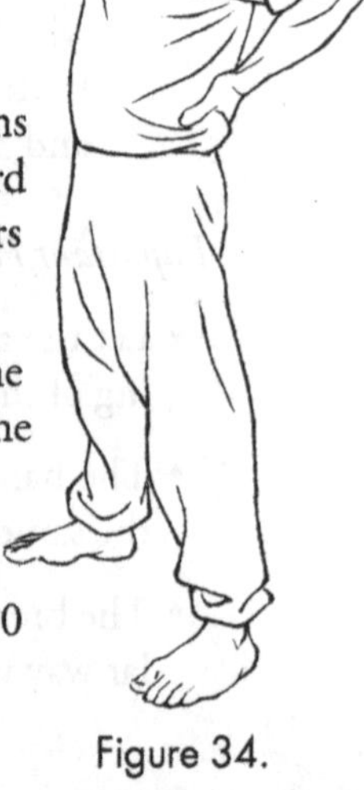

Figure 34.

Important Points

- Keep the movements light and slow.

- Feel how the hip joints open and close as you rotate through the movement.

- Breathe naturally.

- Keep the feet flat on the ground throughout the rotation.

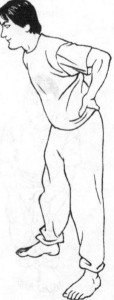

Figure 35.

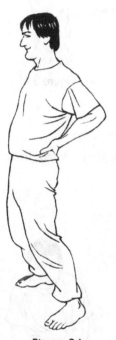

Figure 36.

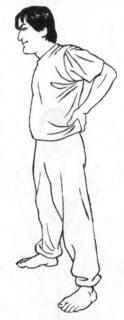

Figure 37.

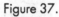

Figure 38.

10: Knee Rotation and Bending

Start: Start with the feet together, knees locked, and your hands on your knees. (Figure 39.)

1. Bend the knees and rotate them in a clockwise circle. (Figures 40–42.) End by returning them to the locked position. (Figure 39.)

2. Repeat 6–10 times.

3. Bend and rotate the knees counterclockwise 6–10 times.

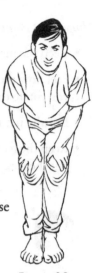

Figure 39.

Important Points

- Move easily and within a range of motion in which the knees are not strained.

- Breathe naturally. Do not hold your breath.

- Let the knees come gently to the locked position. Do not force them.

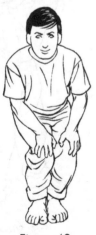

Figure 40.

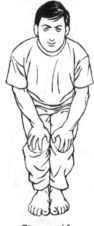

Figure 41.

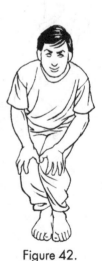

Figure 42.

11: Phoenix Stretch

Start: Start with the heels together and arms at your sides.

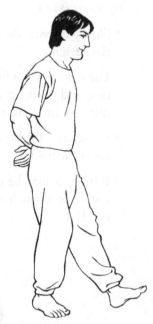

1. Extend the left leg straight out in front, placing the left heel on the ground with the toes pointing upward. The right foot points rightward 45 degrees. Simultaneously, your hands go behind your back, the left hand holding the right wrist. (Figure 43.)

2. Keep the hips facing forward as you exhale and simultaneously lean the upper body forward. (Figure 44.) Allow the chest to fall toward the knee.

3. Hold this position as you slowly inhale and exhale three times, using natural diaphragmatic breath-

Figure 43.

ing. Feel the breath fill the lower abdomen and the lower back. Feel a widening in the lower back area.

4. Inhale and rise slowly.

5. Step the left leg back to the right so that the heels are touching.

6. Extend the right leg out in front, placing the heel on the ground with the toes pointing upward. Repeat on the right leg.

7. Repeat 2–5 times on each leg, alternating legs.

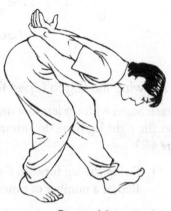

Figure 44.

Important Points

- Slowly increase the range of motion over time without forcing the stretch.

- Use the breath to increase the range of motion, relax the muscles, and open up the back. Visualize that you are breathing into any area that feels tight or restricted.

- Coordinate the breathing with the movement, exhaling as you lower the body and inhaling as you raise the body.

- Initially it may be difficult to do the exercise correctly. Using a stool or a bench may help to control the body weight. (Figure 45.)

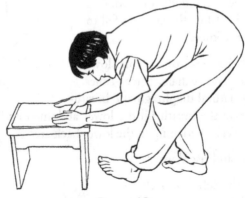

Figure 45.

12: Swing the Leg to Open the Hip

Start: Stand with the left foot on a brick, a large book, or on a step. Let the right leg hang downward so that it can swing freely. (Figure 46.)

1. Swing the leg forward and backward. (Figures 47 and 48.) Repeat a number of times.

2. Switch legs and repeat.

Important Points

- Let the hip joint hang open so that the leg can swing freely.

- Do not force the motion to try to increase the height of the foot during the swing.

- Breathe naturally without holding the breath.

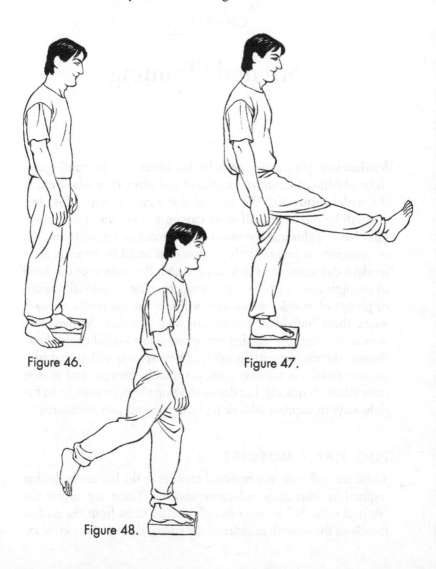

Figure 46.

Figure 47.

Figure 48.

CHAPTER 6

Strength Training

Modern strength training probably has its roots in the training regimen of Milo of Crotona, an athlete and strongman who lived in the sixth century B.C. We are told that Milo developed his great strength by carrying a calf every day until it became a full-grown bull. Free weights and the use of weight machines in which weight or resistance is progressively increased in small increments are a modern-day adaptation of Milo's method. Proponents of this form of strength training believe that strengthening individual muscles or groups of muscles in isolation will increase the body's strength when these individual groups are used together. Studies have shown that strength training can increase joint stability and bone density, thereby preventing injury. There is no question that progressive resistance training increases muscle strength and muscle mass relatively quickly, but does it develop the right muscles in the right ways to improve athletic performance and prevent injuries?

TOO MANY MUSCLES

There are well over four hundred muscles in the human body that respond to conscious voluntary control. These are called the "skeletal muscles," in order to differentiate them from the cardiac muscle or the smooth muscles of the viscera that contract involuntarily. It is virtually impossible to exercise all the skeletal muscles individually. Therefore most strength-training routines tend to focus on the larger, more superficial muscle groups at the expense of many of the deeper, smaller muscles that may be equally important in generating strength and power and maintaining joint stability. The shoulder is a good example of this. Most weight-training routines focus on the larger, more superficial muscles of the shoulder and shoulder girdle—the deltoid, trapezius, and rhomboid muscles—despite the fact that the rotator cuff muscles are responsible for the shoulder's strength during rotation and for maintaining stability through the shoulder's extensive range of motion. The tendons of these four muscles blend with and strengthen the joint capsule. They are critical to functional strength in the shoulder, yet they are rarely addressed effectively in most strength-training routines.

TENDON STRENGTH VS. BULGING MUSCLES

Gains in strength and muscular endurance are often accompanied by an increase in the size of the individual muscle fibers and therefore the girth of the muscle. This increase in size is known as "muscular hypertrophy." It is believed that muscular hypertrophy is regulated primarily by testosterone, which is why increases in muscle mass are more prevalent in men. Many weight-training programs create relatively rapid increases in muscle mass. As a consequence, it is easy to develop bulging muscles that are strong in the belly (middle of the muscle) but relatively weak at the muscle ends (the tendons).

It is a natural tendency when working against a measured resistance to want to see quick improvement. This generally means increasing the resistance. The result is that many people increase the resistance too quickly, causing them to exercise the muscle unevenly through its arc of contraction. This places the focus of the exercise on the muscle belly. A weight that will adequately challenge the muscle belly will be too heavy for the muscle ends to lift using correct form. Modern exercise machines attempt to correct this problem by changing resistance through the arc of the muscle's contraction through the use of levers, hydraulics, or adjustable cams. However, it is difficult to create a machine that will adjust to a wide variety of body types and limb lengths.

Proponents of weight training argue that muscle hypertrophy does not decrease flexibility. Yet we have all seen individuals whose bulging arm muscles prevent the normal swinging of the arms when walking. Contrast this with individuals with long muscles that work smoothly throughout their full range of motion. Is the greater strength of bulging muscles a functional strength that is useful in sports activities or everyday movements?

Strength Relative to the Angle of Contraction

Strength varies relative to the angle of contraction. In the bicep curl shown in figure 49, strength is maximal at 90 degrees but decreases as you move away from ninety degrees. If you could lift 100 pounds at ninety degrees, you might be able to lift only 45 pounds at 180 degrees and, at other points along the muscle's length, 60 to 90 pounds. With most weight machines or free weights, the muscle is not being developed evenly. The weight of 45 pounds will not adequately overload and therefore challenge the bicep muscle at 90 degrees, and the 100-pound weight will be too much for the muscle at 170 or 180 degrees.

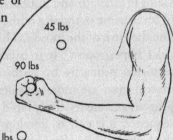

Figure 49.

In general in the West, the tendons are considered to be rope-like extensions of the muscles that do not contract, yet strength exercises are recommended for preventing injury because they increase the stability of the joint. To do this there must be some increased strengthening of tendons and ligaments. In the East, there has traditionally been an emphasis on developing strength and power through natural movements that work the full length of the muscle evenly. The result is a long, smooth muscle that is strong at the muscle belly and the ends of the muscle. This kind of "tendon strength" can generate tremendous power that is not a product of bulging muscles. I will never forget my amazement at the powerful grip of one of my teachers who stood five feet three inches and weighed 120 pounds. At eighty-two, though his arm muscles looked flaccid, he had a grip like iron and could pull me off balance with ease. His strikes, which appeared to be light and weak, penetrated to my bones.

MUSCLES DON'T WORK ALONE

There are few everyday activities in which we employ the strength of a single muscle in isolation. Tests of the strength in isolated muscle groups measure only what they test. They are not indicative of the strength of the whole body. The body is designed to be used as a whole. The more we use the whole body in a smooth, coordinated way, the more efficiently it can function. Kinesiologists (people who study movement) have known for a long time that joints and muscles act in three-dimensional connected chains that wrap the body, crossing from leg and hip to the opposite shoulder and arm. This has been likened to a serape, the Mexican shawl worn over one shoulder and crossing to the opposite hip. In pushing or throwing movements, we tend to generate power from the foot to the opposite hand. As the foot pushes off the ground, extending the hip and knee, the waist rotates and the muscles of the torso accelerate the outward extension of the arm muscles. When we pull or hold something we reverse this process, pulling from the periphery back through the body to the opposite foot. This serape effect is present in most sports activities such as running, biking, tennis, and golf.

Movements requiring strength that are common to sports activities and exercise routines probably derive from the primal actions that we perform as infants, pulling things we want toward us and pushing things we don't want away from us. An infant engages its entire body and spirit in these actions. Efficient employment of strength and power derives from cultivating coordinated whole-body action in these primal movements. Each muscle must contract and relax at the right time. This process can be likened to a series of intermeshed gears. As one turns it sets the others turning.

Learning to use the body this way requires training exercises that program the muscles and the nervous system to respond correctly at the right time. Unfortunately, most weight-training exercises fail to do this. By isolating muscle groups into simple two-dimensional exercises, weight training imprints a segmented type of strength into the neuromuscular system. When I was a personal trainer, I worked with an incredibly strong female athlete. She could pull down and press huge amounts of weight and lift the entire weight stack on many of the machines, but she could not do a single pull-up. It took a month of daily practice before she could do even one. Her strength-training routine simply did not prepare her for the coordinated shifts from one muscle group to another that are required in performing a pull-up.

Having said this, I should add that it is the very isolation of muscles that makes weight-training and other progressive resistance exercises so useful in the *initial* stages of injury rehabilitation. Injured joints in which connective tissue has been torn or overstretched often require specific exercises to strengthen areas weakened by the injury or by inactivity during the healing process. Weight resistance training can also be very effective in cases of chronic injury where specific muscle imbalances need to be addressed. Once the joint regains some stability and the muscles are more balanced in strength, these exercises can be supplemented and eventually replaced by activities and exercises that use the body as a whole. Whole-body exercises help to reintegrate the injured tissue with the rest of the body.

RESISTANCE TRAINING CAN CAUSE INJURY

A significant number of people seen by orthopedists and sports medicine specialists did not injure themselves in sports activities. Their injuries occurred while using exercise machines or weights. In weight training, improvement is measured by increasing the amount of weight. This feeds into our natural tendency to feel that if a little is good, more is better. Usually the injuries are the result of overstrain caused by increasing resistance too quickly or exercising incorrectly. The common tale of many who injure themselves during resistance training is, "I was doing fine, then I added ten pounds and it felt great, but later my arm hurt and I had to stop exercising."

Weight training works by overloading the muscle. This means exercising it against maximal or near maximal resistance. While this does stimulate physiological adaptations that increase muscular size and strength, it can also overload the joint and damage muscles and tendons.

Developing the large, powerful muscles of the body at the expense of the opposing antagonistic muscle groups and the smaller stabilizing muscles can also set the body up for injury. In my opinion, unbalanced muscular development is the cause of many sports injuries. Athletic trainers have become increasingly aware of the tendency to overdevelop the quadriceps muscles. These powerful leg extensors must be properly balanced by the hamstrings, which flex the leg. If overdeveloped, the quadriceps can literally pull the tibia and femur apart, tearing the ACL (anterior cruciate ligament), which stabilizes the knee joint from front to back. Overdevelopment of the quadriceps is also the cause of many pulled and torn hamstrings.

This kind of muscular imbalance can also affect posture, upsetting the body's natural balance. One patient presented me with knee pain that did not respond to acupuncture and massage. He was engaged in a weight-training program that overdeveloped his quadriceps. This caused him to overextend his whole body in standing and walking so that he was tilted forward. These postural changes in turn increased pressure on the front of the knee joint. His trainer recognized the problem and created a more balanced

The Big Three

Three Common Weight Exercises That
Consistently Cause Injury

Some traditional weight-training exercises actually put the body into mechanically weak positions, making it more susceptible to injury. Three exercises in particular consistently cause training injuries:

1. DEAD LIFTS: Dead lifts put the back in a mechanically weak position. This forces you to use the abdominal muscles to prevent pressure on the lumbar discs. Although traditionally used by power lifters to strengthen the back and develop power in the large muscle groups of the back, dead lifts are unsuitable for most athletes because of the potential for injury.

2. SQUATS: Squats are an excellent exercise to develop power in the legs and back. They are part of the Eight Brocade Plus exercises discussed later in this chapter. However, squats against resistance or with a loaded barbell on the shoulders are difficult to do correctly with proper form. They can also overstress the back and the knees. I know of several personal trainers who have herniated discs or aggravated an existing back problem by doing squats. Even leg press machines, which simulate a squat, can be problematic because of the potential pressure put on the lower back. Performed *properly* and slowly, without weights, squats are excellent for developing whole-body power and can actually help those with back pain and herniated discs.

3. MILITARY PRESSES: Military presses, in which the weight is pressed upward behind the head, are the culprit in many neck and shoulder girdle injuries. Although the neck should not be used during this exercise, all too often as the muscles begin to fatigue, the neck tilts forward and the shoulders hunch, putting pressure on the neck muscles and the cervical discs.

program of quadriceps and hamstring strengthening. His posture improved and the pain disappeared.

My own experience working in New York City's elite gyms in the early 1980s was that for many people, weight training fails to live up to its promise. Increases in real applied strength were minimal and often made at the cost of reduced flexibility or injury. In addition, by isolating body parts and exercising them individually, many of my clients were actually prevented from developing the smooth, effortless power that comes from using the body properly as a coordinated whole. These observations led me to further investigate the nature of strength and power and how they can be developed efficiently.

WHAT IS STRENGTH?

In order to better understand how to increase strength, we need to have a concept of what strength is. In general, our tendency is to view strength in terms of quantity. If you have bigger muscles, can lift more weight, do more push-ups, or throw the ball farther, you are considered to be stronger. Yet strength has many facets that are not so easy to quantify. The dictionary defines strength as power, force, vigor, the ability to resist strain or stress, and toughness or durability. Clearly there is more to strength than how much weight you can lift.

Sports physiologists have known for at least a century that strength training is very specific. For it to be effective in relation to everyday actions or athletic activities, it must duplicate the joint angles at which the muscle groups are being used and the type of contraction the muscles need to perform. Isometric exercises, which involve pushing or pulling against a fixed, immovable resistance, are known to produce tremendous gains in strength. However, isometric exercises contract the muscle with the joint at a single fixed angle, so functional strength in the muscle is increased only at that specific angle. For example, contracting the bicep muscle with the arm bent at ninety degrees will increase strength in the bicep only when the joint is at that angle. Since it would be impossible to exercise each joint at every angle, isometric exercises are usually employed in the early stages of physical therapy to increase joint stability or as supplemental training. Weight resistance training exercises muscles and joints through many angles of contraction but often cannot exercise them evenly throughout the contraction and in many cases cannot duplicate the type of contraction that occurs when the muscle is used in an athletic maneuver. Leg extension exercises on a machine are not the same as kicking a ball.

Because strength is so specific to the type of contraction the muscle is undergoing, it is often, for conceptual purposes, differentiated into three subtypes:

1. **Static strength:** The ability to apply or resist a force—for example, the slow lifting of the maximum weight that a muscle or group of muscles can lift.

2. **Power/explosive strength:** The functional application of strength combined with speed. Many sports activities such as sprinting, hitting, or throwing a ball require this kind of strength. It is exemplified by Olympic power lifters, who throw huge weights over their heads in a single explosive motion.

3. **Muscle endurance/dynamic strength:** The ability of a muscle or group of muscles to sustain a static contraction or repeat the same contraction over and over. Most endurance sports require this kind of strength.

Our daily activities and most sports require some measure of all three aspects of strength, yet most strength-training routines develop only one or two of the three. Since most of us have only limited time to devote to strength training, we need something that efficiently strengthens our joints and muscles through their full range of motion and rotation and in the way we will actually use them.

Although Milo of Crotona is viewed by many as the father of modern weight training, in fact he was doing something completely different. Lifting a calf every day and carrying it around is completely different from the isolated muscle training prevalent today. Milo's unique form of strength training employed the power of the whole body and all three types of strength. Moreover, Milo was not just a strongman. His chosen sport was pankration, a brutal, no-holds-barred form of hand-to-hand combat that probably required many different forms of training.

Most experts in exercise physiology would agree that the mechanisms responsible for increases in static strength, power, and muscular endurance are not clear. There is every indication that changes in the neuromuscular system that include both peripheral and central nervous system involvement may be more important than biochemical changes at the level of the muscle and its fibers. Neurological adaptations in the inhibitory control mechanisms (the mechanisms that prevent a muscle from contracting) may well be the keys to strength and power. In other words, the practical manifestation of strength in a given activity may lie in the ability to override the neurological protective mechanisms that inhibit the muscle from contracting or cause the antagonist muscles to contract. These protective reflexes are there to protect joints and muscles from being damaged by the force of a sudden muscular contraction. Often when we try to hit or throw something hard, the result is a clumsy, weak movement, because we have engaged these protective reflexes. When we relax the movement is often powerful and coordinated.

Through their observation of animals in the natural world (see chapter 5), the Chinese gained an understanding of the neuromuscular adaptations that could increase strength. This led them to embrace a very different concept of strength training from that of Western athletes. They saw that the powerful actions characteristic of each animal were not the result of isolated muscles contracting, but a function of the coordinated use of the animal's whole body. Synergistic coordination of the muscles, relaxed deep breathing, and concentrated focus of the spirit and the vital energy allow the animal to bring its maximum strength to bear in a single moment. Nothing inhibits or interferes with the animal's ability to manifest its potential strength.

When animal movements were adapted to create exercises that would improve a human being's ability to actualize the strength of the whole body, they were quickly adopted by martial artists, who saw in them the potential to improve across the board the strength, power, and endurance necessary for combat. The powerful, primal movements of animals inspired many of the martial arts and health exercises that are still taught in China today. Hua Tuo, the famous physician from the Han dynasty, created the "Five Animal Frolics," a set of health exercises developed from studying the movements of the deer, bear, monkey, bird, and tiger in their natural habitat in the mountains of China. Legend has it that the inspiration for the art of tai chi chuan came from watching a fight between a crane and a snake.

These exercises came to be referred to as *nei gong* ("internal exercise") because they develop the body from the inside out rather than focusing simply on the external musculature. The practice of internal exercises develops a refined strength. This refined strength can be likened to crude metal that is gradually transformed into tempered steel. This tempering is achieved through slow, steady movements that exercise the muscles evenly throughout their full range of motion. As you move slowly with focused attention, chains of muscles contract and relax synergistically, without engaging the inhibitory reflexes that can interfere with muscle contraction and reduce the applied force of the body's strength. These internal exercises employ natural movements that use the whole body and have wide applicability to sports and activities that require strength, power, and endurance.

One student who had previously raced mountain bikes out west moved to the city. With no bike to ride, she began to study martial arts. After a year of not biking and practicing internal exercises, she visited her old biking buddies and found not only that she could go faster than many of them, but that she also had more endurance than in the past.

The Eight Brocade Plus exercises are a form of internal exercise, or *nei gong*. They are said to have been created by Marshal Yue Fei, a great hero and martial artist from the Song dynasty. Since that time, they have been used by the Chinese people as a series of health and rejuvenation exercises and by martial arts masters to develop refined strength and power. The Eight Brocade Plus exercises include some variations of the original eight that have been added over the centuries to provide a more comprehensive method of increasing strength and suppleness. If you are in good health and training for sports, the exercises should be performed vigorously.

For rehabilitation they can be done more gently and slowly. For those with injuries to the lower body, the exercises may be done seated, with the exception of number 6.

THE EIGHT BROCADE PLUS

The Eight Brocade Plus exercises can be performed in 20–30 minutes.

The Basics

There are a few things to remember when performing the Eight Brocade Plus:

- The *head* is erect, as though suspended by a thread from the top of the head.

- The *tailbone* drops under, as though attached to a plumb line. This allows a slight bending to occur at the hip joints.

- The *shoulders* relax and drop.

- The *tongue tip* is on the roof of the mouth.

- *Breathe* through the nose, using natural diaphragmatic breathing. Do not force the breath.

- Relax the *chest*.

- The *mind* is fully engaged in the movements, watching and listening to the body.

- *Movements* are slow and relaxed, without any excess tension. It is as though you are moving through a medium like water that provides a constant resistance against every inch of the body as it moves.

- *Repetitions.* There is no fixed number of repetitions for each exercise. The numbers given here are merely general guidelines. More is not necessarily better.

1: Supporting the Sky with Both Hands

Start: Stand with the feet about shoulder width apart and the knees slightly bent, arms at your sides.

1. Inhale as the arms raise to the sides and come overhead, fingertips pointing toward each other. (Figures 50 and 51.)

2. Continue to inhale as you press the hands upward, as though lifting something heavy. Simultaneously extend the hip and knees so that the power of the legs is transmitted through the palms. (Figure 52.) Continue until the arms are fully extended overhead.

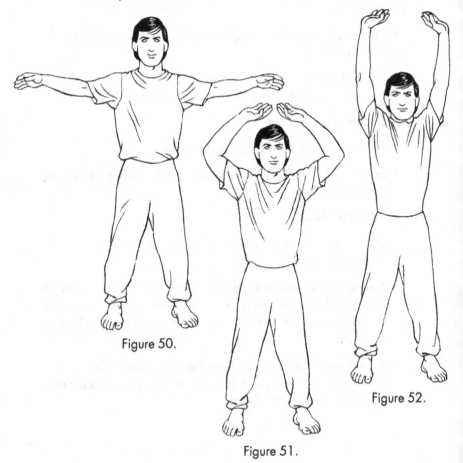

Figure 50.

Figure 52.

Figure 51.

3. Exhale and slowly bend the arms and knees, returning to the position in Figure 50.

4. Continue to exhale and lower the arms to the start position.

5. Repeat 8–10 times.

Important Points

• Keep the shoulders relaxed as the arms push overhead.

• Use the power of the legs to extend the arms.

2: Drawing the Bow to Shoot the Eagle

Start: Stand in the "horse-riding posture," with the legs wider than shoulder width apart and the knees bent. Bend at the hips as though you are about to sit on a low stool.

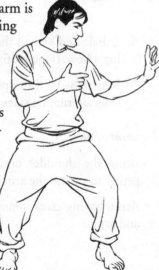

1. Raise the arms so that the left arm is bent with the elbow hanging down and the palm facing to the side. Extend the forefinger and open the space between the thumb and forefinger. The right palm faces the chest as though gently grasping a bow-string with the fingertips. (Figure 53.)

2. Inhale. Then exhale and slowly extend the left arm outward to the side as though drawing a bow. (Figure 54.) Let the shoulder blades move toward each other, thereby separating the arms.

Figure 53.

3. Inhale and smoothly shift the arms to the other side. (Figure 55.)

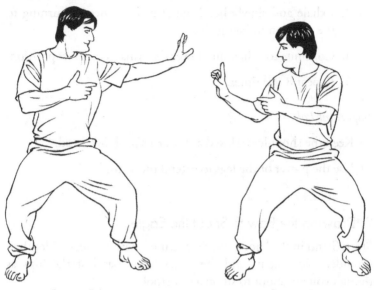

Figure 54.   Figure 55.

4. Exhale and extend the right arm outward as though drawing a bow. (Figure 56.)

5. Repeat 8–10 times per side, alternating sides.

Important Points

• Bring the shoulder blades together to extend the arms.

• Avoid having excess tension in the hands and arms.

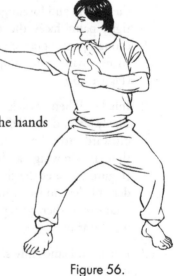

Figure 56.

3: Holding Up a Single Hand

Start: Stand with the feet shoulder width apart and the knees slightly bent, arms at your sides.

1. Inhale and raise the right hand overhead so that the palm faces the ceiling and simultaneously let the left palm fall in front of the left leg, palm down. (Figure 57.)

2. Continue to inhale and simultaneously push the right palm upward and the left palm downward. Extend the legs so that the power of the legs is transmitted into the hands. (Figure 58.)

3. Exhale and bend the arms, bringing them in front of the body as the right palm turns to face down and the left palm turns to face up. (Figure 59.)

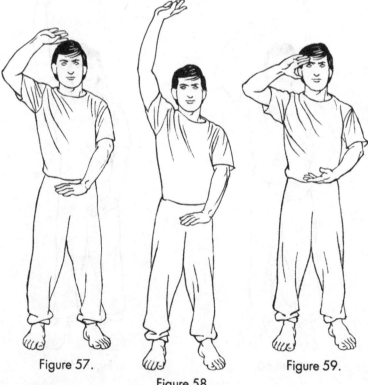

Figure 57.

Figure 58.

Figure 59.

4. As the hands pass each other, begin to inhale until the left palm is overhead facing upward and the right palm is facing downward in front of the right leg. (Figure 60.)

5. Continue to inhale and simultaneously push the left palm upward and the right palm downward. Extend the legs so that the power of the legs is transmitted into the hands. (Figure 61.)

6. Repeat 8–10 times per side, alternating sides.

Important Points

• Coordinate the breath and the movements.

• Let the back muscles be pulled in opposite directions by the movements.

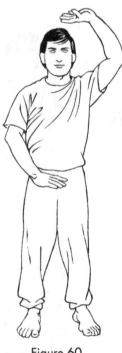

Figure 60.

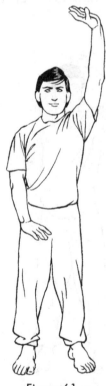

Figure 61.

4: Looking Backward While Twisting like a Dragon

Start: Stand with the feet a little wider than shoulder width apart and the knees bent. The elbows are bent so that the palms face downward at the level of the hips. (Figure 62.)

1. Inhale as you turn the body left and look over the left shoulder. Extend the right leg, pushing off the sole of the foot to shift your weight toward the left leg. Use the turning of the body to arc the hands around you so that the right hand faces outward at the height of the head and the left hand faces outward at the level of the buttocks. (Figure 63.)

2. Exhale and return the body to the start position.

3. Repeat on the other side, turning to look over the right shoulder. (Figure 64.)

4. Repeat 6–8 times, alternating sides.

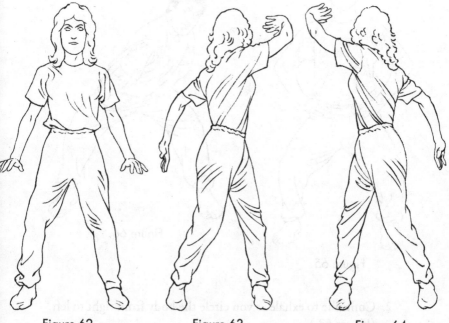

Figure 62.   Figure 63.   Figure 64.

Important Points

- Let the waist drive the arms as they arc around the body.

- Keep the neck relaxed.

- Initiate the turning movement by slowly extending the leg and shifting weight.

5: Shake the Head and Wag the Tail

Start: Stand in the "horse-riding posture" as in exercise 2, but with the hands on the crease of the hips, thumbs facing outward. (Figure 65.)

1. Exhale and lean the body to the right, extending the left arm. (Figure 66.)

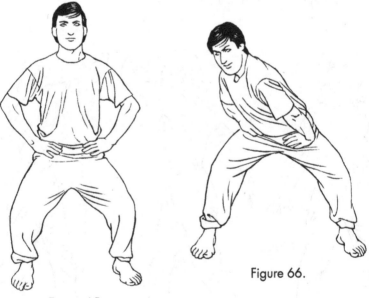

Figure 65.

Figure 66.

2. Continue to exhale as you circle the body from right to left. (Figure 67.)

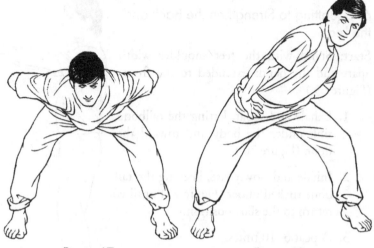

Figure 67.   Figure 68.

3. Inhale as you lean the body to the left, and straighten the right arm. (Figure 68.)

4. Continue inhaling as you sink the tailbone and straighten the body, returning to the start position. (Figure 65.)

5. Repeat circling from left to right.

6. Repeat 8–10 times.

Important Points

• Move slowly and relax the upper body as much as possible.

• Avoid holding the breath.

6: Squatting to Strengthen the Back and the Legs

Start: Stand with the feet shoulder width apart and the hands extended to the front. (Figure 69.)

1. Exhale and squat, letting the tailbone sink under the body and toward the floor. (Figure 70.)

2. Inhale and slowly rise, keeping the tailbone tucked under (Figure 71) until you return to the start position.

3. Repeat 6–10 times.

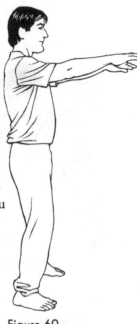

Figure 69.

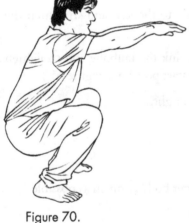

Figure 70.

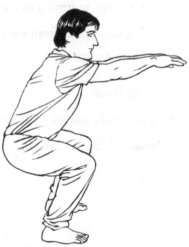

Figure 71.

Important Points

- Move slowly and keep the tailbone tucked under as you lower and rise.

- Keep the feet flat on the floor and the knees over the feet.

- In the beginning it is useful to lightly hold on to a table or bar to aid balance and achieve correct form.

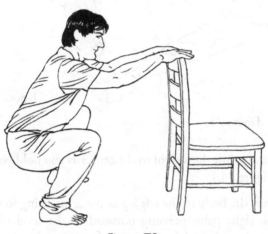

Figure 72.

7: Leopard Crouches in the Grass

Start: Stand with the feet shoulder width apart and your hands at your sides.

1. Step the right foot out to the right as the arms swing to the right, the left palm pressing outward at the level of the right armpit and the right palm pressing outward in front of the left corner of the forehead. Simultaneously, the body squats down on the right leg. Both feet are flat on the floor, and the left leg is stretched straight. The eyes look toward the left, and the waist and hips turn toward the left side. (Figure 73.) Hold this posture for several seconds.

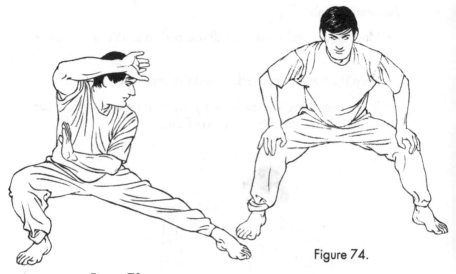

Figure 74.

Figure 73.

2. Slowly shift the weight to the center as you hold your knees. (Figure 74.)

3. Shift the body to the left leg as the arms swing to the right, the right palm pressing outward at the level of the left armpit and the left palm pressing outward in front of the right corner of the forehead. (Figure 75.) Hold this posture for several seconds.

4. Repeat 2–3 times on each side.

Important Points

- Breathe naturally.

- Perform the exercise slowly, focusing on stability and keeping the hips relaxed.

- As you improve, hold the position for longer periods rather than increasing the repetitions.

Figure 75.

• In the beginning it is not necessary to go all the way down into the posture. A chair or low stool may be used to aid in balance. (Figure 76.)

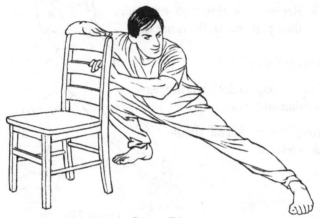

Figure 76.

8: The Black Dragon Enters the Cave

Start: Step the right foot out in a lunge position. The hands rest palm up along the lower ribs with the fingers pointing forward, the elbows are bent about 90 degrees, and the upper body is upright. (Figure 77.)

1. Inhale. Exhale as you push the palms forward and slowly turn the palm centers toward each other. Simultaneously push off the left leg and incline the body forward. At full extension, the palms face downward and the fingers point out away from the body. (Figure 78.)

Figure 77.

2. Inhale and return the body to its original (start) position (Figure 77) by slowly pulling the hands back as you turn them palm up and straightening the upper body.

3. Repeat 6–8 times on one side, then perform on the other side.

Important Points

• Use the legs to drive the arm extension and rotation.

• Keep the neck and shoulders relaxed.

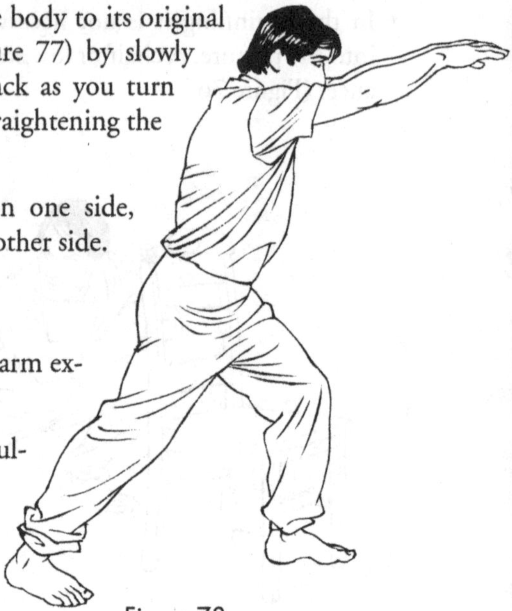

Figure 78.

9: The Prone Tiger Pounces on Its Prey

Start: Take a push-up position on the ground with your feet together and your hands in fists. The buttocks are raised into the air, and the head is down. (Figure 79.)

1. Exhale and lower the chest toward the ground (figure 80), then push up with the arms, leaving the buttocks down so that the head rises upward to the front. (Figure 81.)

2. Inhale and lower the chest back to the ground (figure 82), then raise the buttocks as you push back with the arms to the start position. (Figure 79.)

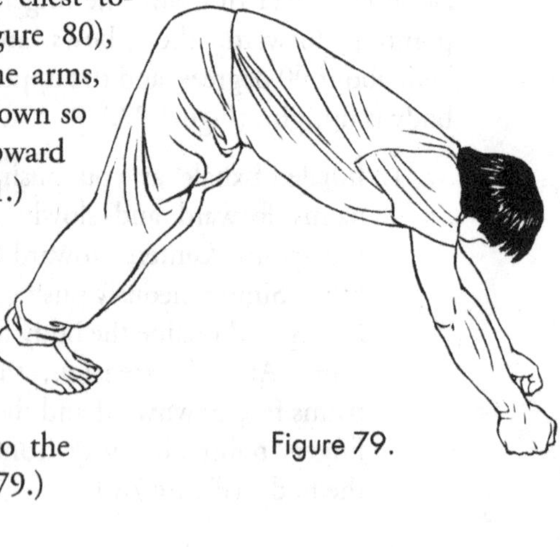

Figure 79.

3. Repeat as many times your endurance permits, up to 15 times.

Important Points

- Regulate the breath so that it is smooth, even, and unrestricted on the inhale and exhale.

- Keep the elbows slightly inward so that they brush the ribs as you push outward and as you pull back to the start position.

- Concentrate the mind and spirit throughout the exercise.

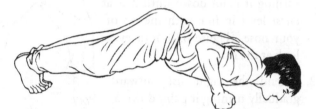

Figure 80.

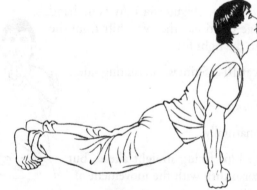

Figure 81.

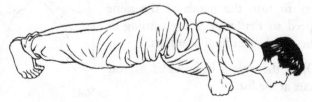

Figure 82.

10: Clenching the Fists and Glaring Increases Strength

Start: Stand in the "horse-riding posture," with the legs wider than shoulder width apart and the knees bent. Bend at the hips as though you are about to sit on a low stool. The hands are in fists, palm up at the level of the lower ribs.

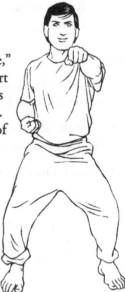

Figure 83.

1. Extend the left fist out, gradually turning it palm down until it is at chest level in line with the tip of your nose. (Figure 83.) Your eyes look at the fist.

2. Extend the right fist outward, gradually turning it palm down as you simultaneously rotate the left fist palm up and withdraw it back to your hip. (Figure 84.) As your hands change positions, the eyes shift from the left to the right fist.

3. Repeat 10–15 times, alternating sides.

Important Points

- Breathe naturally.

- Keep the hips facing straight ahead, but let the torso turn with the movement of the arms.

- Try to turn the hands at the same speed so that they finish turning as they reach their final positions.

- Open the eyes a little wider as you stare at the fist.

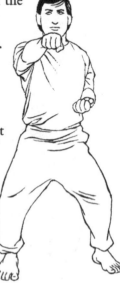

Figure 84.

11: Shaking the Body Wards Off Illness

Start: Stand with the feet shoulder width apart and the backs of the hands on the lower back. (Figure 85.)

1. Shake the body up and down by bending slightly and straightening the knees.

2. Repeat 8–10 times.

Important Points

• Breathe naturally.

• Keep the body relaxed, and avoid using excessive force.

12: Embracing the Moon

Start: Stand with the feet shoulder width apart and the knees slightly bent. Let the tailbone fall under. The hips should be bent slightly as though about to sit. Raise the arms until they are just below shoulder height, with the fingers pointing at each other. The fingers are slightly separated. Feel as though you are embracing a large ball. (Figure 86.)

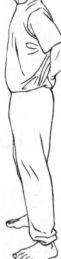

Figure 85.

1. Hold this posture for 1–10 minutes. Start with 1 minute and increase the time as desired.

2. To finish, slowly lower the hands, stand quietly, and attend to the breath for 1 minute.

Important Points

• Breathe naturally, attending to but not forcing the breath.

• Relax the shoulders. Feel as though the arms are suspended by strings or buoyed up by balloons.

• Let the weight settle evenly into the soles of the feet.

Figure 86.

CHAPTER 7

Diet and Health Maintenance

DIET

The great doctors of ancient China regarded exercise and diet as the highest forms of medicine because they had the potential to increase a person's vital energy and prevent disease from taking root in the body. Today most people would argue that a healthy, balanced diet is an important ingredient in maintaining health and vitality. But what is a healthy diet? Rather than having *an* answer to this question, we have too many answers. For years, we were told that low-fat diets were better for us. Now carbohydrates are the culprits, and eating fat can actually prevent obesity, while carbohydrates simply make us hungrier. We are told to choose foods according to our blood type, or to eat more protein or more foods containing omega-3 fatty acids. Some people say that foods in the nightshade family, like tomatoes, are terrible, while others point out that tomatoes can help prevent prostate disorders. Some experts warn against the evils of alcohol consumption. Others extol the health benefits of drinking a glass of wine or two a day. We are not supposed to eat too many dairy products like cheese, yet somehow it is okay for the French. We are told to be vegetarians, eat more fiber, drink less coffee (although it turns out coffee contains many antioxidants), try fish oil, drink green tea, drink more water, take vitamin supplements. The list goes on and on. We know more about foods then we have ever known before, yet we are more confused than ever about what to eat.

This absurd situation is the result of attempting to break down whole foods into their component parts, in order to understand how they work, and our tendency to divide foods into good and bad categories. It is the nature of science to break things down into their component parts. Breaking foods down into their nutritional components has made it possible to understand diseases caused by nutritional deficiency. What this paradigm does not tell us is the amount of these nutrients needed for optimal health and performance. It is impossible to construct a diet by dividing food into nutritional packets, because these food components do not exist alone in nature. They are part of a whole. Isolating a chemical compound that prevents prostate problems is not the same as eating a tomato and may not work effectively. Science knows much that is useful, but it has yet to construct a pill that can replace eating whole foods. People who are sick or injured need to eat whole foods that are rich in nutrition to give their bodies the energy to heal.

Our tendency to moralize about foods and divide foods into good and bad categories also adds to our confusion and leads us into unhealthy eating habits. No food is a priori good or bad. It is always a question of how much that food is eaten and who is eating it, in addition to how it is balanced against other foods that are being consumed. No one particular diet is correct for everyone. A vegetarian diet that is perfect for one individual may be disastrous for another.

Red meat is viewed by many as unhealthy, and certainly overconsumption of red meat can contribute to health problems, yet our bodies need the concentrated energy and proteins that animal meat supplies. It is difficult to get these from other food sources. I have observed that many vegetarians need to eat constantly throughout the day to make up for the deficit created by their diet. Tofu is generally considered to be healthy. It is often argued that it is a primary protein source and staple of the Asian diet. However, tofu and soy products actually form only a small part of the Asian diet, and overconsumption of soy can cause a buildup of mucus and phlegm. There is also evidence that too much soy can lead to hormonal imbalances.

One should be wary of restrictive diets that eliminate entire food categories, such as starches and carbohydrates, or fats, or proteins. Often all they accomplish is the creation of a nutritional imbalance. I have seen several people who went on no-fat diets quickly develop strange neurological symptoms. When they went back to eating some fat, the symptoms disappeared. The body needs fat to protect our internal organs and build myelin, a fatty substance that forms a sheath around nerve fibers. Without fat these structures cannot function properly.

It is tempting to want to divide foods into good or bad categories, because it makes the whole question of what to eat seem much simpler. We get the added benefit of feeling virtuous because we have exerted our will and avoided the "bad" foods. However, this kind of thinking seems silly when we consider the diversity of foods eaten across the planet by healthy people. Moral judgments about food often cause people to cling to unhealthy eating habits that are not working for them. Obsessional judgments about food are usually much more damaging than the foods themselves. Chinese medicine recognizes that excessive worry, overthinking, and obsessing about food can actually interfere with and damage the body's ability to digest and assimilate food.

Athletic endeavors and recuperation from injury require proper nutrition. We all know how to eat properly, but we have forgotten how to trust our own instincts. Unless a scientific study or some diet or nutritional expert confirms the efficacy of a food, we feel it might not be good for us. We have become separated from our common sense.

Commonsense Eating

1. **The basis of proper nutrition is whole, natural foods that are as fresh as possible.** It is not just a question of eating the right number of grams of protein or carbohydrates. What is important is the specific kinds of proteins and carbohydrates we ingest and how fresh and chemical-free they are. The fresher and less processed the food, the more life force

it contains. Avoid chemically processed foods and foods containing chemical additives and preservatives. They are harder for the body to break down and assimilate and usually provide less nutrition.

2. **Eat a diverse and balanced diet.** This is not as complicated as you may have been led to believe. The diet of healthy peasant people from almost any ethnic background is usually fairly balanced, supplying them with enough nutrients to do hard physical work on a daily basis. The ancient Chinese were a practical agrarian people. Look at the average Chinese meal. There are several dishes, often with small amounts of meat. There are vegetables and spices cooked with the meat and often side dishes of cooked vegetables, root vegetables, bean curd, nuts, and pickled vegetables. There might be grains such as rice or millet, or noodles made from wheat, millet, or rice. Often soups are served with the meal, and in northern China, where it is colder, the soups are thick and nourishing. Every culture seems to naturally solve the problem of combining and balancing foods, often by simply serving a wide variety of grains, legumes, soups, meats, vegetables, fruits, nuts, and spices all within a single meal. Home-cooked meals I had growing up as an Italian American included many or all of these foods. Only in modern culture do we consider a Coke, hamburger, and fries a meal.

3. **Include foods that tonify the qi and blood.** These are the foods that most nourish the body. The Chinese have studied foods for centuries. Lengthy treatises have been written about the healing properties of food and dietary dos and don'ts in relation to a host of injuries and diseases. In Chinese medicine, the inherent medicinal properties of foods are analyzed in much the same way as the properties of medicinal herbs. Foods that nourish qi and blood are important staple foods found in the diets of many cultures. These foods are particularly important to have in your diet when recovering from an injury, because they provide damaged or overused tissues with the nutrients they need to heal. Foods

that nourish qi and blood tend to be nutritious foods such as meats and fish, root vegetables, leafy greens, nourishing grains, eggs, dairy products such as milk and butter, and some nuts and dried fruits. The following list is not by any means exhaustive, but it will give you an example of the foods that are considered to tonify the qi and the blood.

Oatmeal	Yams	Liver
Millet	Potatoes	Tuna
Rice	Corn	Catfish
Many grains	Carrots	Salmon
Dates	Spinach	Goat
Milk	Many leafy greens	Oyster
Pumpkin	Cooked peaches	Shark
Raisins	Eggs	Warming spices
Longan fruit	Sea cucumber	that aid
Beets	Turnips	digestion:
Eel	Tripe	cardamom,
Sugar, maple	Pork	ginger, cin-
syrup, and	Mutton	namon, and
honey (small	Beef	nutmeg (small
amounts)	Chicken	amounts)

4. **Don't obsess about what you eat.** Eat a variety of foods and enjoy them as much as possible. It is not always possible to eat perfectly all the time. The ability to eat a wide variety of foods allows us to better adapt to the outside world. Worrying too much about what you eat can actually interfere with digestion and assimilation.

A Balanced Diet

In addition to eating a wide variety of foods, there are several other ways of thinking about food that can help you to eat a more balanced diet.

1. **Balance the five flavors:** Foods can be classified according to their tastes or flavors. These flavors indicate not only

what something tastes like on your tongue, but the inherent qualities of foods that have certain traits and produce certain effects. In addition, each flavor "homes," or is drawn, to one of the viscera.

Sweet Foods

Sweet foods supplement the qi. Many of the nourishing foods that tonify the qi and blood (see list) are sweet in nature. This is because they home to the organs of digestion—the spleen, pancreas, and stomach. These foods not only activate, but provide nourishment to the internal organs and the muscles, bones, tendons, and ligaments. The activating quality of sweet foods is why sugar, candy, and other sweets give us a momentary energy lift. While a little sugar can nourish the qi, in general refined sugar and sweets are empty of nutrition and cannot sustain the body's energy. Although nourishing sweet foods supplement the body's energy and replenish fluids, they have a rich, thick quality that can be cloying and lead to stagnation of body fluids if they are overindulged in and not balanced by the other flavors.

Bitter Foods

Bitter foods home to the heart. Bitter vegetables like watercress, leeks, mustard greens, and asparagus stimulate the heart. They help the body eliminate heat and can disperse stagnant moisture and qi. However, in excess they can be drying or can overstimulate the heart. Coffee is a good example of a bitter food that strongly stimulates the heart and lungs. It moves the qi, which is why we feel a "lift" after drinking a cup. Coffee also moves stagnant moisture (a cup of espresso helps you feel less bloated after a heavy meal) but is also a diuretic, therefore in excess can be too drying.

Pungent (Spicy) Foods

Many of the spices we use to flavor food are considered to be pungent. Some examples are garlic, ginger, marjoram, basil, nutmeg, and various kinds of pepper. These foods home to the lungs. They tend to warm the body, thereby accelerating the movement of the qi and blood (circulation). Therefore, such foods tend to disperse stagnant moisture or congealed blood. Pungent foods also promote sweating, which helps to release excess heat from the body. They tend to be very strong, which is why they are usually used in small quantities to spice up food. In excess pungent foods can exhaust the qi by moving it too quickly. Spicy foods can also overheat the body and dry the tissues if eaten in excess.

Sour Foods

Sour foods such as vinegar, mustard, liver, yogurt, and many fruits home to the liver and gallbladder. While pungent foods promote sweating, sour foods can slow or arrest perspiration. Many fruits are both sweet and sour. Their sweet nature makes them moistening and thirst-quenching, while their sour nature tones the viscera, muscles, and sinews because the sour flavor tends to astringe the tissues. Think of how sucking on a lemon makes your mouth pucker up. In excess this astringent aspect of the sour flavor can cause muscles and sinews to tighten and cramp, causing pain and restriction.

Salty Foods

We associate salt with the sea, and in fact, many salty foods come from the sea: shellfish, seaweed, many ocean fish, and, of course, salt itself. Salt has a powerful effect on the fluids of the body. Concentrations of salt can pull fluid across cell membranes. Because the kidneys are the primary filter of body fluids, the salty taste is said to home to the kidneys. Salty foods tend to concentrate qi, blood, and fluids and move them downward toward the lower body, aiding the kidney function. We tend to forget that many fast foods, processed and canned food, and even soybeans contain salt. These foods should be consumed in moderation, because in excess salty foods can cause stagnation and retention of fluids.

A diet that includes all of the five flavors ensures that the qi and blood are properly nourished and flowing and that the functions of the internal organs are harmonious and balanced. It is also clear that preference for one flavor over the others can lead to an imbalance. While it may seem complicated to balance the five flavors, in fact it is simply a question of being aware of their properties and including a little of each taste in every meal or at least in your daily diet. You will find that a meal that includes all five tastes is usually very satisfying and energizing. Many people who have tried eating this way notice that they tend to snack less, because the meal left them with a feeling of fulfillment and satisfaction.

2. **Balance hot and cold foods:** While the five tastes describe the inherent traits of foods, hot and cold are a way of expressing their energetic nature. In this context, hot and cold refer not only to the temperature of a food, but to an intrinsic energy that the food itself contains. Hot foods like lamb or cinnamon are intrinsically warming and stimulating. In excess they cause a buildup of heat in the body that dries out the tissues and can damage the blood. Cold foods act to cool, calm, sedate, and relax. In excess they can be hard on the body's digestive system, which must first warm up the foods in order to break them down and assimilate the nutrients. In Chinese medicine, it is said that too many cooling foods put out or weaken the digestive fire, akin to putting out the fire under the cooking pot. While hot-natured foods activate the blood and qi, too many cold foods will stagnate or constrict the movement of the blood and qi.

   The temperature at which food is eaten is also part of this equation. Iced foods and drinks cool the body, and hot foods are more activating. Broiling or roasting imparts more heat, while steaming or poaching are milder forms of cooking that add less heat. Sushi is an interesting example of trying to balance hot and cold foods. Raw fish, especially shellfish, is very cooling. Eating sushi with warming condiments like ginger and wasabi to some degree counteracts the cold nature of the fish. In addition, since many vegetables are cool in nature, cooking them lightly warms them so that they are more easily digested and their nutrients more easily assimilated.

HOT FOODS	WARM FOODS
Many spices, including cinnamon, cayenne pepper, and chili peppers	Beef
	Coffee
	Poultry
	Root vegetables
Lamb	Onions and scallions
Dried ginger	Fresh ginger
Spirits	Wine and beer

COLD FOODS	COOL FOODS
Most shellfish	Pork
Carp	Lettuce
Many river fish	Dairy products
Tomatoes	Mushrooms
Seaweed	Cucumber
Celery	Radish
Watermelon	Most fruits
Bananas	Soy
Tea	

NEUTRAL FOODS	
Fish such as shark, salmon, catfish, and tuna	White sugar
	String beans
Eggs	Carrots
Bread	Most grains and legumes
Corn	Most nuts

3. **Balance heavy and light foods:** Simple and light diets have been recommended by generations of Chinese physicians to preserve good health. In the seventh century, Sun Si-miao, one of China's most famous physicians, advocated a diet that stressed natural light foods like cereals, grains, beans, vegetables, and fruit. An excess of heavy, greasy, rich foods often results in a buildup of heat, dampness, and phlegm. Too much heavy food can also overload the stomach, causing food to stagnate and ferment in the stomach, leading to belching and gas. Interestingly, in both the Far East and the West, heavy foods tend to be the feast foods,

eaten on special occasions and holidays. This does not mean that heavy foods are bad or should not be eaten on a daily basis, just that they must be moderated by a larger amount of light foods. If you already glanced at the list that follows, you might have noticed that the heavier foods are in general more warming and the lighter foods more neutral and cooling, so just balancing heavy and light foods tends to create a balance of hot and cold foods as well.

HEAVY FOODS	LIGHT FOODS
Alcohol	Fruit
Bread	Grains
Dairy products	Cooked vegetables
Deep-fried food	Potatoes
Fish	Sprouts and salads
Meat	Beans and legumes
Desserts	Nuts

Foods That Prevent Injuries from Healing

The intrinsic nature of certain foods may make them unsuitable for consumption when you have a sports injury. These foods should be temporarily eliminated from your diet or strictly limited while the injury is still healing.

COLD FOOD

Cold foods slow the healing process. They tax the available energy by drawing on it to warm the food for assimilation. Cold causes contraction and coagulation, obstructing circulation and blocking the flow of qi and blood. Therefore, cold foods should be avoided with sinew injuries and in the earlier stages of fractures. Cold-temperature foods such as iced drinks, ice cream, and fruit juices are particularly harmful, but foods that are classified as cooling, such as shellfish, raw vegetables, and fruits, should also be avoided or limited until the injury heals. One common mistake that many people make is to eat large amounts of raw vegetables and fruits or juiced vegetables and fruits. Cooked vegetables are far more nutritious than raw vegetables. The cell walls of plants are incredibly strong and difficult for the human digestive system to break down. Cooking vegetables breaks down the nutritional components bound up in the cells of plants so that they can easily be absorbed and assimilated by our digestive systems. Rather than "eating healthier," people who consume too many raw foods tax their digestive system and risk impairing the normal circulation of blood and qi.

SOUR FOOD

Sour foods home to the liver. The astringent nature of sour food tends to tone the sinews because of the liver's relationship with the sinews. This can be important in helping to restore the integrity of overstretched tendons and ligaments. However, in the early stages of sinew injuries, especially when using soaks and liniments that restore circulation and relax spasms in the soft tissue, sour foods are contraindicated. Their action of astringing and tightening the sinews can contribute to cramping and pain. Although we tend to think of fruits as being sweet, most fruits are also considered to be sour in nature, as well as energetically cold. Intake of fruits should be reduced when one is recovering from a tendon or ligament injury. I have seen numerous cases in which a simple dietary change resolved a tendon or ligament problem where other therapies failed. One of my students had resumed running after a layoff of a year or more. He was young and healthy, but after several weeks his knee started to bother him. Structurally everything was fine, yet two acupuncture treatments failed to make any improvement at all. When I quizzed him about his diet, he told me he drank a quart of iced orange juice first thing in the morning. This large amount of a sour, cold food before his morning run was causing the tendons in his knee to cramp and tighten. When he eliminated the juice from his diet, the pain stopped.

Before you start cutting out sour foods altogether, remember that the sour flavor also acts to tone or give integrity to organs and soft tissue; therefore, they are a necessary part of a balanced diet. In fact, sour foods can be beneficial in cases where the tendons and ligaments are overstretched owing to chronic or repeated injury, thereby endangering the integrity of the joint. The traditional Chinese dietary therapy for this situation is beef tendon cooked with vinegar. An alternative, recommended by one of my mentors in Chinese sports medicine, is beef adobo cooked with tomatoes and vinegar. Beef nourishes the muscles and sinews, while the tomatoes and vinegar help to astringe the soft tissue. Common sour foods include

Barbecue sauce	Buttermilk
Fruits—most	Fruit juices
Lemons (very sour)	Tomatoes
Vinegar	Pickles/pickled vegetables
Sour cream	Yeast
Yogurt	Liver (any kind)
Sourdough bread	Salad dressings
Salami	Mustard

SPICY FOODS

Spicy foods can help move stagnant blood and qi and move the circulation. Because they accelerate the circulation and push it toward the surface of the body, they should not be eaten in cases of injuries with large open wounds or after surgical procedures.

SHELLFISH

Shellfish tend to be cold and therefore restrict circulation and contribute to coagulation of blood and fluids. Their consumption should be restricted when there is an injury to the sinews. However, there is another problem with shellfish. Even the more nourishing shellfish such as oysters or mussels are traditionally prohibited when one is recovering from a sinew injury because they are considered to contain a toxic element that interferes with the healing process. Although modern research has not substantiated the existence of such a toxin, in my clinic I have seen several people who did not recover completely until they stopped eating shellfish. Once the injury is fully healed, shellfish can be consumed safely again.

Controlling Fluid Intake

Daily consumption of liquids is essential to replace the fluids we lose every day. In general, drinking six to eight cups of liquid, including soups, is enough to replenish lost fluids. If you are exercising or working in the heat, you need to drink more. As a culture we tend to drink too many fluids. Fluids do not "flush out" the system. Fluids must be processed and pushed out of the body by the kidneys and bladder. Excessive intake of fluids strains the ability of the kidneys to process them. This drains the kidney energy, which the Chinese consider to be the root of the body's energy. Coffee, tea, and diet drinks (particularly colas) act as diuretics, which cause more frequent urination, thereby making us thirstier, so that we need more fluids, which further overstrains the body.

Although we need fluids to moisten tendons and ligaments so that they are supple and strong, overconsumption of fluids can actually impair the healing process, by draining the kidney energy and impairing circulation through fluid retention. Cold drinks are particularly damaging, as the cold also impairs circulation, further depleting the body's energy. I have seen several patients develop strange pains in the knees and feet. They were all drinking several thirty-two-ounce diet sodas a day, which over-taxed and depleted their kidneys. In Chinese medicine, pains in the lower legs and feet are often related to an insufficiency of kidney energy. Usually, normalizing fluid intake will rectify these types of problems.

Nutritional Supplements: Help or Hindrance?

The best way to get enough vitamins and minerals is through eating a wide variety of whole foods. However, when you are injured or engaged in activities that push you to the limits of your strength, endurance, and flexibility, nutritional supplements can help you to heal faster and prevent injury. Extra nutrition can be particularly important for individuals taking anti-inflammatories or blood pressure medication. Many drugs deplete nutrients, and it is not always possible to make up the deficit only through eating whole foods.

Despite their benefits, vitamins and minerals that have been isolated from foods are strong medicine and should be taken carefully and selectively. Many people advocate high dosages of vitamins and minerals that are difficult or impossible for the body to process. Rather than promoting optimal performance, they deplete the body and further tax its resources, as it must now either store or excrete these unnecessary substances. These problems can be avoided by following a few simple rules:

1. **Take vitamins in reasonable dosages of 300–400 mg.** Many people take excessive amounts of vitamins. The water-soluble B and C vitamins are excreted in the urine if they cannot be absorbed. This leads to increased urination, which forces the kidneys and bladder to work harder, again draining the body's energy. Some vitamins and minerals cannot be excreted so easily. There is evidence that excess intake of calcium can lead to hypertension, kidney stones, and calcifications throughout the body and that too much zinc can contribute to high levels of cholesterol, while excessive amounts of iron in adults may contribute to heart disease. Since even the experts cannot agree on dosage levels beyond the minimum daily requirements, it is safer to take lower dosages of vitamins and minerals. Remember, they are supplements, not replacements for proper nutrition.

2. **Dosages of vitamins and minerals should be balanced.** Many vitamins and minerals need to be taken with other specific nutrients to be absorbed properly or to work effectively in the body. To be used properly, calcium needs to be taken with vitamin D and balanced by magnesium, while vitamin C needs to be balanced by bioflavonoids, the pigments that accompany vitamin C in plant foods. These nutrients are naturally balanced in foods but may not be in a vitamin pill. The simplest and safest way to supplement your diet is to find a balanced multivitamin that gives you low dosages of essential minerals and vitamins.

3. **Take vitamins and minerals derived from natural rather than synthetic sources.** There is every indication that vitamins and minerals that are derived from natural sources are easier to assimilate and more potent than their synthetic counterparts.

Chinese Herbs

Herbal medicines have been taken for centuries in China. Chinese herbs have withstood the test of time—they are used all over the world to treat an amazing variety of illnesses. Many medicinal herbs like ginger or cardamom are also used in cooking. Others like yam root are basically nutritionally concentrated foods. These herbs tend to have mild, safe actions with little chance of side effects. However, the bulk of the herbs that make up the Chinese materia medica are powerful medicines that can be combined into thousands of herbal formulas. Martial artists have traditionally used herbs to optimize athletic performance and promote health and longevity. Ma huang (ephedra) was taken by the imperial guards so they could stay awake through the long night watches, while ginseng and astragalus were prized as restorative tonic herbs. Today, many of these herbs are included in vitamin pills or in "energy" drinks. Ginseng and astragalus are sold at every neighborhood store, because of their reputation as adaptogens, herbs that help the body adapt to stress.

Herbs are medicines. They can be abused even by knowledgeable people. Ma huang does help you to stay awake, but it does not "give you energy" any more than caffeine does. Ma huang accelerates the movement of qi and blood and acts as a diaphoretic and bronchial dilator. In Chinese medicine, it is traditionally used in conjunction with other herbs for asthma, bronchitis, pneumonia, and arthritic conditions. Taken alone or in diet pills, it can seriously deplete the body's energy. Ginseng and other tonic herbs like astragalus and tang kuei are usually included in herbal formulas that combine a number of herbs to create a particular synergistic and balanced action in the body. These kinds of herbs are not appropriate for everyone to take indiscriminately. When taken alone as tonics, they can cause problems with digestion and circulation.

My friend and colleague Mr. Huang Guo-qi is a lecturer at the Shanghai College of Traditional Chinese Medicine. He frequently sees patients who overindulge in tonic herbs like ginseng. Mr. Huang feels that "in general the problem caused by excessive intake of tonics is an excess pattern. Too much has been taken into the body and accumulated. If the problem is due to ginseng, there is often a feeling that food is not digesting or that the stomach is full. There may be a stuffy feeling in the chest or acid regurgitation, belching or poor appetite, and even nosebleeds or bleeding from the gums."

Sports injuries are often accompanied by stagnation of qi, blood, and fluids. Taking tonic herbs without first removing this stagnation can actually make the problem worse by increasing the stagnation. It is akin to throwing more logs on a beaver dam (see chapter 3). The blockage must be removed before the system can be tonified.

Many people want tonifying herbs like ginseng because they feel they need more energy. All too often they are like a friend of mine who came to see my mentor in herbal medicine. He worked two jobs, slept four hours a night, ate on the run, and drank twenty cups of coffee a day. He felt tired and wanted tonic herbs to give him more energy. We tried to explain to him that although herbs would give him more energy, he would be burning the candle at both ends, depleting the body's resources even more quickly. He went away rather dissatisfied with the two of us. My friend is an extreme example, but for many busy people, lifestyle changes such as eating well and getting sufficient rest will be of more benefit than tonic herbs. Beyond the specific tonic herb formulas discussed in this book, if you feel that you need tonic herbs, you should see a professional practitioner of traditional Chinese medicine. He or she can find or create a formula that is suitable for your condition and constitution.

Fasting, Liver Detoxification, and Colon Cleansing

In general, Chinese medicine does not advocate fasting or frequent detoxification regimes because these practices tend to deplete the body's vital energy. In the West, many alternative health practitioners advocate periodic detoxification of the liver and colon, in order to purge the body of toxins. If you are going to try a detoxification program, it should be undertaken carefully and infrequently because it places additional stress on the body's energy. Many detoxifying herbs are cooling and dispersing in nature. They not only eliminate toxins but also tend to disperse the body's vital energy. Fasting also stresses the body, forcing it to operate on stored nutrients. These kinds of cleansing programs should be undertaken infrequently, no more than once a year, as part of a well-thought-out, *short-term* plan that includes dietary modifications. Because fasting, liver detoxification, and colon-cleansing programs make demands on the body's reserves, they should not be undertaken when trying to recover from an injury, while training hard, or during the competitive season.

Today many people take colon cleansers such as cascara sagrada (a purgative) and psyllium seed husks (these seeds provide fiber, which expands in the intestines and helps to push out stuck fecal matter) with herbs such as dandelion and curcuma that disperse heat from the liver. Often their daily routine includes megavitamins and tonic herbs as well. This is counterproductive. The concentrated nutrients found in herbs and vitamin pills cannot be absorbed and assimilated if the liver and colon are being cleansed and dispersed at the same time. One young man I was treating for sports injuries complained about digestive problems and lack of energy. An herbal formula aimed at harmonizing his digestion produced minimal results. Then he told me about the number of herbs and supplements he took daily. In addition to megadoses of vitamins and minerals, he was taking a number of tonic herbs, antioxidants, colon-cleansing formulas, and liver-detoxifying herbs. I had him eliminate all but a multivitamin, an experiment he was eager to try, as it would save him several hundred dollars a month. Within two weeks his digestion improved and he began to have more energy.

For those who feel that detoxification and cleansing are important health-enhancing procedures, following is a simple, safe detoxification diet:

One-Week Detoxification Program

Undertake this program only when you are not ill or recovering from an injury. Pregnant women, nursing mothers, and children should not fast or undergo detoxification programs.

Detoxification should be done during a period when you will be getting sufficient rest, are not training hard, and are not under physical or emotional stress. Furthermore, do not undertake a detoxification program even under these conditions more than once a year.

On day one, fast for twenty-four hours and drink only water and fresh fruit and vegetable juices. Then, on days two through seven:

- In the morning on an empty stomach, drink 2–3 tablespoons of a mixture of equal parts lemon juice and olive oil.

- Eat as much of the following foods as you like: grains, cooked vegetables, fruits, legumes, potatoes, nuts, and yogurt.

- Eat small portions of meat or fish once a day.

- Eat no more than two or three pats of butter per day, and use only one or two pinches of salt per day.

- Drink only fresh water or room-temperature fruit juices or vegetable juices.

- Avoid activating, warming spices like peppers, cinnamon, mint, cardamom, and ginger.

- No alcohol, tea, or coffee. Herbal tea is fine as long as it does not contain any of the spices just listed.

- You may use minimal amounts of sugar or maple syrup in cooking.

- Cook foods lightly, preferably by steaming, poaching, or stir-frying. Do not eat broiled or deep-fried foods.

- Use light oils like olive or safflower for cooking.

Afterward, slowly return to your normal diet, gradually adding heavier, richer foods, coffee, and tea over several days. Avoid the tendency to immediately have all your favorite foods and desserts.

LIFESTYLE AND HEALTH MAINTENANCE

Balancing Work and Rest

Balancing work and rest is very difficult in the modern world. Many of us work fifty hours a week. In our time off there are social events to attend, bills to pay, chores to do around the house, and recreational activities that keep us mentally and physically engaged during our leisure time. It is important to realize that every thought, action, and movement is a manifestation of our vital energy. We need time to recoup our energy, particularly when injured. This often means not doing so much and taking time off to just "be." Scheduling this quiet time on a daily or weekly basis allows the body to replenish its resources and to divert some of these resources to healing. When you are recovering from a sports injury, enjoy your time off from your favorite activities. Realize that a little rest now may mean you will get back to playing sooner.

Adapting Athletic Training and Exercise to the Seasons

The ancient Chinese were an agrarian people who survived by learning to harmonize the body's energies with the energies of the world around them. They noticed that seasonal changes were accompanied by changes in the movement of their own vital energy and that by adapting their lifestyle to nature's cycles, they could live longer, healthier lives. These practical methods of adapting daily life to seasonal changes gradually became part of Chinese medicine. Over time, martial arts masters also adopted these ideas. They found that if they trained their bodies in accordance with the cyclical changes of the world around them, they achieved better results, reduced injuries, and prevented illness. In modern times, though many of us live in cities and have the benefit of central heating and climate-controlled environments, our bodies still feel the pull of nature's rhythms. Today's athletes have much to gain by understanding these simple principles of healthy living discovered by the ancient Chinese.

In spring and summer, the energies of the earth grow and flourish. This is the time to train hard and push the body. Stretching and strengthening exercises should be performed in the spring and summer when the weather is warm and the muscles are ready to be taxed. Let the body perspire, to release excess heat.

In the fall, as the energies of the earth pull inward, you should slowly taper off from hard training, gradually reducing your exertion as the weather grows colder. In the winter, plants and animals are more dormant, replenishing their energies for the spring. Human beings too should conserve their energy. This is the time to work more on athletic skills and techniques and to do lighter, more inward-directed exercise such as yoga, the Daily Dozen, or the Eight Brocade Plus. Sweat less to retain the body's heat and prevent wind and cold from penetrating muscles and joints.

To understand and use these ideas, we must remember that they are guidelines, not hard-and-fast rules. Obviously the competitive season for many sports is in the winter, so taking it easy might not be an option. However, it is still prudent to cut back on other, less necessary activities to conserve the body's energy. For example, I treated a young man who played professional tennis matches in the winter. On his off time he entered in ski-racing competitions for fun. Despite being young and in good health, he was unable to heal his injuries from the competitive season because he was pushing his body too hard at a time when it needed to replenish its energies.

Certain climates are warm all year round, so it might seem unnecessary to adapt one's lifestyle to the seasons, but even in warmer climes there are seasonal changes that our bodies respond to. I spent months studying martial arts in the Philippines, where the weather is hot and sultry most of the time; but in the monsoon season, when it rains every day and the air is cooler, we relaxed our training a bit to allow our bodies to adjust to the cooler temperatures.

With central heating and air-conditioning, we are more buffered from the elements than were the people of ancient China. However, we are still subject to the effects of seasonal change on our body's energy. Many people even in cities feel the urge to sleep longer and rest more in the winter and to be more active and stay outside later in the summer. Moreover, artificial climate control can actually create climatic illness out of season. Each summer I see several people who develop painfully stiff necks caused by sleeping with the air-conditioning blowing on them, a condition that in ancient China occurred only in winter.

Sex, Health, and Athletic Performance

In Chinese medicine, sex is viewed as a healthy and natural expression of the body and mind. Sex is, in and of itself, neither good nor bad; rather, it is our relationship to it that can be either health enhancing or harmful. Too little sex can result in diseases of accumulation or stagnation, while too much can deplete and exhaust the body. In particular, ejaculation in men is considered to exhaust the reproductive essence stored in the kidneys. These energies, referred to collectively as the *jing*, are easily replaced by young men but become harder to replace as men age and the vital energy declines.

The *jing* forms the root of the body's energies. *Jing* nourishes the bones, which are associated with the kidneys, and forms part of the blood, which nourishes the internal organs and all the tissues of the body, including the tendons and ligaments. We sometimes draw upon the *jing* in moments of extreme exertion or when we tax our endurance to the utmost. Ancient Taoists practiced methods of sexual yoga to replenish the *jing* and promote longevity. While these practices are complex and tied in with Taoist mysticism, some of the basic Taoist concepts about sex are worth considering, as they have proven themselves clinically over hundreds of years and are part of Chinese medicine as it is practiced today. The Taoists advocated less frequent ejaculations as a man aged and even went on to propose exactly how often this should be at each respective age.

Since the strength and resilience of men of equal age can vary greatly, it is best to use the following criteria. If you are fatigued and experience a feeling of weakness for some time after sex, or feel that your athletic performance is affected by having sex the night before a sports event or exercise session, then you may be ejaculating too frequently. Traditionally, in injuries such as fractures or torn ligaments it is recommended that sex be curtailed or reduced during the early period of healing so that the body's full energies can be directed toward the injured area. This is particularly important in cases of injury to the knees, the lower back, or the bones, all of which have a direct relationship to the kidneys and therefore to the *jing*. One young man who studied Chinese medicine with me told me that his chronic back and knee pain disappeared when he stopped masturbating every day.

Women also consume *jing* during sex and orgasm, but to a much lesser extent than men, so that pacing sex and the frequency of orgasms seems to be much less critical for women. What does consume *jing* in women are multiple pregnancies, especially those pregnancies that occur in the late thirties and early forties, prolonged breast-feeding, and excessive bleeding during menstruation.

Health Preservation Exercises

One of the great "secrets" of the *nei jia* ("internal") schools of martial arts are some form of health preservation exercises. Although no one knows who created these exercises, they are mentioned in Chinese medical texts as early as the seventh century. These exercises consist of a simple form of self-massage that can be done in a few minutes each morning. Their purpose is to gradually lead the body's energy into balance over a period of time. Although simple in appearance, they are based upon a deep understanding of the internal workings of the human body and the ways in which disease can penetrate the body's defenses. The health preservation exercises stimulate the natural healing powers of the body while preventing disease from taking root. Like many self-cultivation methods, the health preservation exercises produce results through consistent practice over a period of time. The standard recommendation is that one should practice the exercises daily for a period of one hundred days (three months) to see results.

For the athlete, these exercises can be an indispensable tool. Balancing the energetic pathways of the body is critical to prevent injury and illness. Often the factors that set the body up for injury or allow disease to penetrate the body start with minor energetic imbalances. Rebalancing the body on a daily basis is one of the most efficient ways of being proactive, while energizing the body and improving mental focus. One of my patients who does the health preservation exercises daily finds them enormously helpful in reenergizing the body when traveling or when he has to put in extra hours at work. He told me that when he feels his ability to concentrate slipping, he pauses to perform some of the exercises and feels his mind immediately grow clear. Although they can be performed any time throughout the day, the health preservation exercises are usually performed first thing in the morning while lying or sitting in bed. The number of repetitions is based on Chinese numerology, in which nine or multiples of nine are believed to be yang numbers, associated with the heavenly influences that help to dispel earthly accumulations and imbalances. The numbers are merely guidelines for starting out. Later you can do the number of repetitions that feels right for you.

Before starting the exercises, take a few moments to calm the mind. Sit or lie comfortably and breathe slowly, letting the lower abdomen expand with the inhalation. If thoughts come to mind, observe them and let them pass on.

1. Click the teeth together 9 times. Then circle the tongue behind the upper teeth, producing saliva. Swish the saliva in your mouth and then swallow it in 3 parts. Imagine each part traveling down the midline of the body to the area below the navel. There, imagine the saliva transforming into steam, like water hitting a fire. Imagine that the steam expands outward to fill and warm the lower abdomen.

2. Rub the hands together to warm them. Then use the sides of the thumbs to massage downward from the center of the eyebrows and down along both sides of the nose 9 times.

3. Use the fingertips to massage around the eyes 9 times.

4. Wash the face with the palms 9 times.

5. Use your fingertips to "comb" your hair from the front of the forehead to the base of the skull 9 times.

6. With your fingertips, massage the points at the base of the skull. (Figure 87.)

Figure 87.

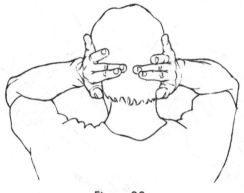

Figure 88.

7. Beat the Sky Drum: Cup the palms over the ears with the fingers touching at the base of the skull. Put the index fingers of each hand on top of the middle fingers. Now flick the index fingers off the middle fingers so that the fingers drum on the base of the skull. (Figure 88.) Repeat 18 times.

8. Massage the ears. There are reflex points in the ear that relate to every part of the body. These are detailed in chapter 13.

9. Use your palms to massage in alternation down the front of your throat 9 times.

10. Rub the right side of the chest with the left hand 9 times. Rub the left side of the chest with the right hand 9 times.

11. Turn the left arm palm up and stroke down the front of the left arm from the shoulders to the fingertips with the right palm. (Figure 89.) Then turn the left arm palm down and stroke up the back of the arm from the fingertips to the base of the neck with the right hand. (Figure 90.) Repeat 9 times. Then repeat 9 times on the other side.

12. Massage the left and right ribs 9 times.

13. With both hands stroke upward from the lower ribs to the solar plexus. Then with the hands touching, stroke down the midline of the body to the pubic bone 9 times.

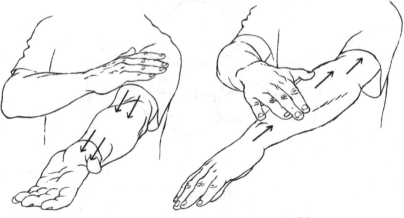

Figure 89.   Figure 90.

14. Put one hand on top of the other and massage below the navel in a circle 36 times clockwise and then 36 times counterclockwise.

   • If you suffer from constipation, massage only in a clockwise direction. This follows the direction of the movement of the intestines and aids elimination.

   • If your stools tend to be loose or you have diarrhea, massage only counterclockwise, as this aids absorption.

15. Put the palms on the back and stroke upward from the sacrum to the kidneys 18 times.

16. Massage the sacrum and the tailbone with the fingertips 9 times.

17. Rub the knees with the palms, circling outward 9 times and inward 9 times.

18. With the palms, massage the KID 1 acupuncture point on the sole of each foot 81 times. (Figure 91.) Rubbing this point, the first point on the kidney meridian, helps to stimulate the kidneys.

Figure 91.

19. Stand. Massage with the palms down the back of the legs from the hips to the feet and then up the inside of the legs from the feet to the abdomen. (Figures 92 and 93.) Repeat 9 times.

20. Relax and breathe for a minute before beginning your day.

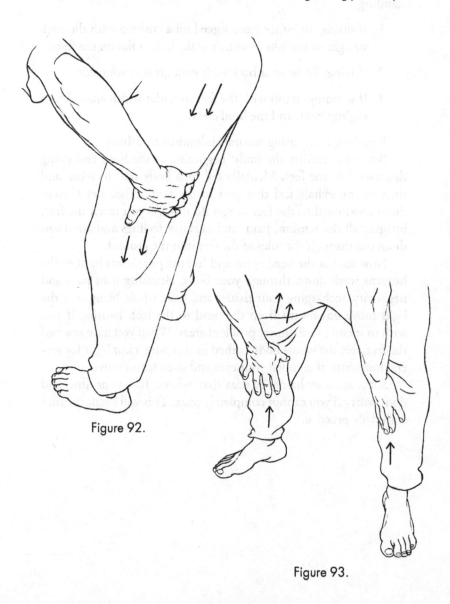

Figure 92.

Figure 93.

Healing Meditation

An ideal time to do this meditation is after the health preservation exercises. Find a comfortable position. It can be sitting, lying, or standing.

1. If sitting, sit either cross-legged on a cushion with the back straight or upright in a chair with the feet flat on the floor.

2. If lying, lie on your back with your arms at your sides.

3. If standing, stand with the feet shoulder width apart, knees slightly bent, and the head erect.

Breathe quietly, using natural abdominal breathing.

Begin by relaxing the body, beginning at the head and going downward to the feet. Mentally tell each body part to relax, and then as you exhale feel that part of the body relax. Let tension drain downward to the feet as you do this. As you reach the feet, imagine all the tension, pain, and negative feelings and emotions drain out through the soles of the feet into the ground.

Now start at the head again and feel the pure, clear light of the heavens wash down through your body, cleansing it of pain and negativity, recharging your tissues and your whole being. Let the light move downward from the head to the feet, pausing if you wish to spend more time at problem areas. When you have reached the feet, feel the whole body bathed in this pure, clear light for several moments, then open your eyes and stretch and move.

Some areas are harder to relax than others. Take your time, and don't worry if you cannot completely relax. This will become easier with daily practice.

The Therapies of Chinese Sports Medicine

INTRODUCTION TO PART III

THE FOUR PILLARS OF CHINESE SPORTS MEDICINE

I Health Preservation

- Diet
- Exercise
- Physical therapy
- Health preservation exercises
- Lifestyle modifications

II Physical Medicine

- Cupping
- Bleeding
- Acupoint stimulation
- Self-massage
- Moxibustion and heat therapy

III External Herb Therapy

- Poultices and plasters (*gao*)
- Liniments
- Herbal soaks

IV Internal herb therapy

- To break up accumulations of qi, blood, and fluids.
- To drive out and disperse accumulations of cold, wind, and damp.
- To stimulate the body's natural healing response and to strengthen sinews and bones.

From the preceding list, it is easy to see that Chinese sports medicine employs a wide variety of therapies to treat sports injuries. This is because no one therapy is suitable for every injury or every individual. Often, multiple therapies are required to return the athlete to optimal health and performance. Because Chinese sports medicine views the human body as an interconnected whole, different therapies can be used to address different parts of the particular condition being treated, thereby resolving the condition more quickly.

Out of this fundamental idea, Chinese medicine developed the four pillars. Traditionally, Chinese doctors learned to use the four pillars through long apprenticeships with master physicians skilled in all aspects of Chinese medicine. You don't need to apprentice with a Chinese doctor to treat your own injuries, but you do need to know about the different treatment modalities that Chinese sports medicine makes available to you.

This section of the book will discuss individual therapies in depth. If you have been reading the book from beginning to end, then you have already read about the first pillar in chapter 7, while chapters 3 and 4 detailed how the four pillars can be integrated to treat tendon and ligament injuries or fractures. Part 4 puts it all together by telling you how to treat your specific injury using all of the four pillars.

Whenever possible, treat your injury with *all* of the four pillars. When you engage the natural healing powers of your body on several levels, it responds more quickly, shortening healing time and preventing reinjury.

CHAPTER 8

Cuts and Lacerations

Cuts and lacerations not only accompany many sports injuries, they are the one trauma injury most of us will suffer repeatedly throughout our lives. Because most wounds are not serious or life threatening, we tend not to worry too much about them. Washing the injured area with soap and water, then applying an antibacterial cream and a clean Band-Aid usually suffices. If the wound becomes infected, there are always antibiotics. Anything more serious can usually be handled by Western medicine, which is extremely effective with serious bleeding injuries. However, we don't want to run to the doctor for a prescription for antibiotics every time we get a deep cut or puncture wound. Although antibiotics are one of the wonders of modern medicine, their progressive overuse in our culture has led to a host of health problems and ever stronger strains of antibiotic-resistant bacteria. Embrace any opportunity to avoid using them. Save them for when you really need them. Fortunately, Chinese sports medicine has a lot to offer for the treatment of wounds. It gives us a first aid for cuts that is more than just putting on a Band-Aid. It can help wounds heal faster, with less scarring and without the need for antibiotics.

The battlefield medicine of ancient China included herbal pills, powders, and salves effective in stopping bleeding, healing wounds, and preventing infection. The Shaolin monks preserved many herbal formulas designed to treat injuries from spears, swords, and other edged weapons. Many of these are still in use today, but the most famous and effective formula of them all is yunnan paiyao.

YUNNAN PAIYAO

Yunnan paiyao is the best all-around formula to stop traumatic bleeding and prevent infection. It is a must for your medicine cabinet or first-aid kit. The ingredients that make up yunnan paiyao were a secret, kept by only one family of doctors. The Communist government forced the family to give up the formula, and it became the property of the state, which made it available cheaply in a variety of forms. Yunnan paiyao was part of China's aid to Vietnam during the Vietnam War owing to its effectiveness in treating battlefield injuries.

Yunnan paiyao both stops bleeding and removes blood clots. These two seemingly contradictory actions are what make it so suitable for healing wounds. As the bleeding stops, blood congeals in the wound. This congealed blood sometimes blocks normal circulation and prevents the wound from healing properly. Yunnan paiyao stops the bleeding but simultaneously encourages normal circulation, removing pus and congealed blood, which can prevent the flesh from being properly nourished. This helps the flesh to regenerate with minimal scarring. Yunnan paiyao is a prepackaged "patent remedy" that comes in two forms:

1. In a small box containing a vial of white powder. A small red pill (see "The Red Pill") is wrapped in the cotton wadding. The powder is easier to apply externally.

2. In a box containing blister packs of 16 capsules each with 1 red pill per blister pack. The capsules are easier to take internally, although they can be broken open so the powder inside can be applied directly on the wound.

Internal Use

Yunnan paiyao can be taken internally if there is suspicion of internal hemorrhage or to prevent and stop infection. In these cases, ¼ teaspoon of powder or 2–3 capsules can be taken with warm water twice a day. This can be useful for head injuries where there may be bruising or bleeding of the brain. In these cases, it is very important to stop any bleeding that may be occurring, while preventing the formation of blood clots that may cause problems later. In instances where there is suspicion of concussion or internal bleeding, take yunnan paiyao and go to the hospital immediately.

For bruises and contusions, sprains, and strains, *where there is no hemorrhage or concussion,* yunnan paiyao is taken with alcohol (vodka or rice wine). In Chinese sports, medicine alcohol is said to "course the channels" by dilating the blood vessels and pushing energy through the meridians. This accentuates yunnan paiyao's property of dispersing stagnant blood. In cases of hemorrhage or concussion, yunnan paiyao should *not* be taken with alcohol.

The Red Pill

The red pill that accompanies each blister pack of capsules and each vial of powder is to be taken only for serious injuries such as stab and gunshot wounds. For this purpose, it is taken with strong rice wine or vodka. I cannot say that I have used the red pill, but martial arts practitioners in China have reported using both it and the powder to heal these kinds of wounds without recourse to antibiotics. I am not recommending that you treat gunshot or stab wounds yourself, but having access to medicines that could save your life is always useful.

External Use

In cases of open wound or infection, yunnan paiayo is very effective when applied directly to the wound. If the wound is bleeding, sprinkle the powder into the wound and use the standard first-aid procedures of direct pressure and elevation of the injured area to stop the bleeding. One of the few times when ice is useful is with wounds where the bleeding won't stop. This is not uncommon with head wounds. When my son's skateboard hit his nose and cut the side of it deeply, local swelling kept the blood from congealing. I daubed yunnan paiyao on the cut and used direct pressure and ice to stop the bleeding. Then we cleaned the cut and applied a paste made from yunnan paiyao under a Band-Aid. The cut healed quickly, with no scar.

Once bleeding is stopped, clean or irrigate the wound and then make a paste with your own saliva and pack the paste over and around the wound. Although water can be used to make the paste, your own saliva contains enzymes that kill bacteria. Finally, cover the wound with a clean bandage. Reapply the yunnan paiyao twice daily until the wound closes. In cases of suppurating wounds, it is better to just sprinkle the powder over the area rather than making a paste, because the wound must dry out in order to heal. A friend of mine had a growth removed from her groin area. Even after two weeks and antibiotics, there was a round, open wound with angry red edges oozing pus. Initially I had her clean the wound, sprinkle yunnan paiyao powder over the area, and cover it with a bandage twice a day. When the wound dried out and started to heal, she made a paste of saliva and powder and applied it twice daily for several weeks. The wound gradually filled in, with minimal scarring.

Yunnan paiyao can be applied as a paste for many kinds of open and infected wounds, including ingrown toenails that have become infected. I have used it with spider bites where the flesh was beginning to die from necrosis. Simultaneous internal and ex-

IMPORTANT!

Yunnan paiyao and all *of the other herbal formulas presented in this book cannot be taken* internally *by pregnant women, as these formulas can be harmful to the fetus.* Blood-activating, stasis-removing formulas disperse accumulations of qi and blood. The fetus is obviously a healthy accumulation that should not be dispersed.

ternal use of yunnan paiyao helped the flesh to regenerate. Often with ingrown toenails or fresh spider or centipede bites it is useful to first apply a paste of water and the green clay used for facials. Leave the clay on for several hours. It will draw the toxins and pus from the area. Then clean the area and apply the yunnan paiyao paste. For more on insect bites, see part 4.

Yunnan paiyao can also be a useful tool in postsurgical healing. Even the less invasive arthroscopic surgical procedures used so widely today create trauma inside the body that is slow to heal, despite the small scars on the surface. The dual actions of yunnan paiyao—stopping bleeding and dispersing stagnant blood—make it ideal for postsurgical use. Generally it is best to wait 2 or 3 days after surgery before taking yunnan paiyao. Then take 2 capsules 2 times a day for a week. One of my patients was undergoing a hip replacement. She took yunnan paiyao for a week after the surgery, followed by several weeks of herbs to move stagnant blood and increase blood circulation to her legs. She also received acupuncture and massage around the hip area and later over the scar. Within days, she was walking well and her healing process was quick and uncomplicated.

AVOIDING STITCHES

Stitches are often a necessity for large wounds, but with some smaller wounds where the skin is thin, particularly those on the face, stitches can be avoided by using the membrane on the inside of an eggshell. Stop the bleeding and clean the wound. Sprinkle yunnan paiyao into it and then close it gently with your fingers as you apply a small piece of the membrane inside an eggshell over the wound. Take half an eggshell and crack the edge of it. Then peel away a small piece of shell. This will usually result in a small piece of the membrane protruding over the edge of the shell. Gently peel a section of the membrane away from the shell.

As it dries, the membrane will draw together the edges of the wound. Leave it for several days. It will either fall off by itself or you can wet it with a damp cloth to make it come off. The wound should now be a closed thin red line. Put yunnan paiyao paste over it for several more days to help it heal quicker. One of my students got hit just below the eye with a heavy wooden staff during a demonstration. The edge of the weapon opened up a gash below her eye. I used exactly the procedures just described to close and heal the wound. This was followed by applications of pearl powder (see "Preventing Scarring"). What promised to be a nasty scar healed, showing only a nearly invisible white line.

PREVENTING SCARRING

Treating open wounds correctly is the best way to prevent scarring. Yunnan paiyao alone helps the flesh regenerate and prevents the complications of blood stasis and infection that can lead to scarring. However, there is more that can be done once the wound is closed but the scar is still active—that is, it is still red and tender. Apply pure pearl powder (made from real pearls) by making it into a paste with your saliva. Often I prefer to mix it with lemon juice because of its astringent, drawing action. Cover with a bandage and reapply several times a day while the scar is healing. Pearl powder helps closed wounds heal with minimal scarring. Pure pearl powder, like yunnan paiyao, is a prepackaged patent remedy available from most Chinese pharmacies and many companies that distribute Chinese herbs.

NOSEBLEEDS

Nosebleeds are usually minor injuries that stop fairly quickly. Sometimes they are hard to stop, particularly following a very hard, direct blow to the nose. Nosebleeds can also be caused by internal factors, such as excess heat driving the blood faster, pushing it out of its normal pathways. It is not uncommon for women to get nosebleeds with their period or for pregnant women to get frequent nosebleeds due to the extra blood in circulation during pregnancy. Nosebleeds caused by internal imbalances require diagnosis and treatment by a professional practitioner of traditional Chinese medicine, but the techniques used to stop nosebleeds caused by trauma will often work to stop the bleeding.

Two acupoints on the hand are useful for stopping nosebleeds. They can be stimulated by taking a piece of string or a shoelace and wrapping it around your hand just below the knuckles. (Figure 94.) Then make a fist to tighten the string around your hand. (Figure 95.) This pressure will often slow or stop the bleeding within 10 or 20 seconds.

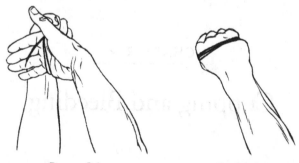

Figure 94.   Figure 95.

Alternatively, tugging hard on the small hairs at the nape of the neck can also help to stop nosebleeds. These methods don't work all the time, but they do work often enough to be worth knowing. They can be used in conjunction with tilting the head back, applying direct pressure, and filling the nose with cotton to speed up clotting.

For unstoppable nosebleeds:

1. Take yunnan paiyao internally.

2. Use the acupoints just mentioned.

3. Stuff the nose with cotton, tilt the head back, and apply direct pressure by gently pinching the nose.

4. Use ice for several minutes to temporarily reduce the swelling and slow the flow of blood.

If a nosebleed caused by a hard blow to the head won't stop, and particularly if it is accompanied by dark, thick blood, it is worth a trip to the doctor to see if damage was done to the cranial bones behind the nose. If the nose is crooked or broken, it should be set by a doctor as soon as possible.

CHAPTER 9

Cupping and Bleeding

When I tell patients they need cupping and bleeding, they usually look nervous and say, "That sounds medieval." In a sense they are right. Cupping and bleeding are therapies that have been around for centuries and are still used in Eastern Europe today. Many Italian grandmothers remember being cupped and bled for colds and stiff necks by their own mothers and grandmothers, and it was a service offered in barbershops in Europe even into the twentieth century. Cupping, a therapy in which a vacuum is created in a glass cup to draw stagnant fluids up to the surface tissues, was such a common therapy among German Jews that the Yiddish expression "That's about as much use as cupping a dead man" became a way of describing something as useless. Although cupping has largely fallen out of fashion in the West, bloodletting is actually used with some frequency in modern medicine. Syringes are often used to drain swollen joints, and leeches have been reintroduced into modern medicine. Leeches are used in conjunction with microvascular surgery and limb and tissue reattachment to prevent postsurgical congestion of the veins and blood clots.

I have found cupping and bleeding to be extraordinarily effective for reducing swelling from sprains and strains or for draining toxic swellings. I have used these techniques effectively on thousands of people and taught them to hundreds of students of Chinese medicine. They are an important stage 1 treatment for many sinew injuries. Cupping and bleeding are safe and easy to perform, having their roots in the "folk medicine" of the villages of ancient China. They later became a part of traditional Chinese medicine as it is practiced today because no other therapy could duplicate their effectiveness.

BLEEDING

Although bleeding can be used to treat a wide variety of conditions, in sports medicine it is used primarily in conjunction with cupping to reduce swelling and draw stagnant blood out of the superficial tissues in the injured area. Bleeding generally conjures up unpleasant images of leeches or overweight aristocrats being bled by court physicians, but bleeding in Chinese medicine means using a small lancet to let out a few drops of blood. Traditionally, a sharp surgical tool called a "three-edged needle" was used to draw blood, but for our purposes a simple sterile lancet that can be found in any drugstore will do the job. These are the same lancets that diabetics use to prick their fingers to test blood sugar levels. The technique is simple. In an injury like a sprain that is inflamed and swollen, make several shallow punctures around and in the swollen area and then apply cups to draw out congealed blood and fluids. Often only a small amount of blood is drawn out of the area. The idea is not to drain the area, but to ease the pressure. This often immediately reduces some of the pain and restores some of the natural movement of the joint.

CUPPING

Cupping is a simple, direct method of pulling stagnant qi, blood, and fluids out of or away from an injured area. When used in conjunction with bleeding, it draws stagnant fluids and blood out of the injured area. When used alone, it draws stagnation up to the surface, where it can be dispersed by massage and local application of Chinese herbs. Cupping is performed by creating a vacuum in a glass cup, thereby drawing skin and muscle tissue up into the cup.

Cupping and bleeding are often a very important first step in the treatment of acute sprains and strains. These methods are particularly useful right after an injury occurs, when the injured area is swollen and discolored, because blood and fluids have accumulated, blocking normal circulation. For example, with a freshly sprained ankle that is swollen and black and blue, bleed the swollen area by making several shallow punctures and then apply cups. Often, the blood that is drawn out into the cup will be quite dark or even black, especially if you are treating the ankle a day or two after the sprain occurred. Once the darker, coagulated blood is drained, bright red, healthy blood will be drawn into the cup. Remember, you are taking out only a small amount of the blood that is pooling outside the blood vessels in the soft tissue. This is the first step in breaking the dam of stagnation blocking normal circulation in the injured area. Cupping and bleeding help to relieve pain by acting like a pressure valve, literally "bleeding off" the excess pressure created by the accumulation of blood and fluids. When combined with massage, herbal therapy, and liniments and poultices, cupping and bleeding can greatly reduce healing time.

Another important use of cupping is in the treatment of poisonous bites or stings from scorpions, centipedes, wasps, and spiders. Toxins from bites and stings can severely damage muscle and nerve tissue. Cupping can be used to draw out the poison. I was bitten on the calf by a spider when mowing the lawn. The bite ached and itched the next day, but I didn't really take notice of it until the ache began to move up my leg toward the knee. The path of the pain and swelling corresponded exactly to the bladder meridian, which runs down the back and through the calf muscle. As the pain approached the top of the calf, I realized that soon it would reach an acupoint behind the knee where the meridian dives deep into the body and connects with the internal organs. I immediately bled the hard area around the bite and applied a cup to draw out the toxin. Then I mixed green clay and water to make a poultice, which I spread thickly over the bite. The clay created a drawing effect, which gradually pulled the swelling back down my leg to the area where I had been bitten. I applied cups one more time the next day. This further reduced swelling around the bite. By the next day, my leg was normal.

Cupping in cases of poisonous bites is always done over the site of the bite. This draws the toxins out at the point of entry. Using a lancet to bleed the hard area around the bite and then applying cups helps facilitate the drawing action of the cups. This should be followed by applying a poultice of green clay mixed with water. This poultice can be left on for several hours or even overnight. As the clay hardens it draws the toxins out of the wound.

Green clay, a beauty product normally used to draw impurities out of the skin, is sold in many drug stores. If the bite is on the face, just apply the clay. Cupping should not be performed on the face. See "Cupping Indications and Contraindications," page 170.

Cupping Methods

There are basically two kinds of cups:

1. **Plastic or glass cups with built-in valves:** These usually come in sets of 10 or 12 cups with a pump. The pump connects to the valve and is used to draw air out of the cup, creating a vacuum. As the air is pulled out, skin and superficial muscle tissue are drawn up into the cup. To remove the cup, open the valve at the top with your fingers and slowly let air back in. This releases the suction. Care must be taken when using this kind of cup in conjunction with bleeding to avoid getting blood in the valves, which are difficult or impossible to clean out. The advantage of this type of cup is that 1 or more can be applied quickly and easily and the amount of suction is easily adjusted.

2. **Glass or bamboo cups:** Specially shaped cups are available from Chinese pharmacies for this purpose, but it is possible to use any small glass with a thick lip so that the edge of the cup does not pinch or cut the skin. I have found that shot glasses or baby food jars tend to work best. In this method, fire is used to create a vacuum by consuming the oxygen in the cup, which is then placed quickly on the skin. This method is sometimes referred to as "fire cupping." To remove the cup, press on the skin along the edge of the cup,

thereby letting air into the cup and releasing the suction. *Never attempt to just pull the cup off the skin.*

There are a number of ways to perform fire cupping. I find the following two to be the easiest and safest:

1. Take an alcohol swab or a piece of gauze dipped in alcohol and hold it firmly with forceps or tweezers. Light the swab on fire, then quickly put down your match or lighter and pick up the cup. For 1 or 2 seconds, hold the cup over the flame so that the tip of the flame is just inside the cup. Then quickly place the cup on the skin. When you place the tip of the flame just inside the mouth of the cup, you must hold the cup close to the area to be cupped so that you can set it on the skin before the air rushes back in, breaking the vacuum. *Important:* Be careful to hold the cup so that the tip of the flame goes just inside of it. If you heat up the lip of the cup, you can cause a burn when you place it on the skin. Be careful with the flame. It is easy to forget about the hand holding the flaming alcohol swab when you are placing the cup. Keep it away from your body and anything flammable (such as your hair), and blow it out immediately after placing the cup. This method is quick but requires the right equipment and a bit of practice. Sometimes it must be repeated several times to get the right amount of suction.

2. For the second method, you need a cup, a coin the size of a quarter, and a small, 2-by-2-inch square of paper toweling. Twist the paper around the coin so that the bottom is flat and the twisted toweling points up. Place it on the skin and light the end of the toweling on fire. The coin creates a buffer between the skin and the flame. When the flame gets going, cover the coin and the surrounding skin with the cup. The fire will go out as the air in the cup is burned up. This creates a vacuum and sucks the flesh up into the cup. The coin is left inside the cup, so this method is not as elegant as the previous one, particularly if you are using cupping together with bleeding; however, this method has the advantage of needing no special equipment.

Cupping often creates a large, circular-shaped bruise that may remain for several days afterward. This is nothing to be alarmed about and is normal when there is stagnation of blood and fluids in the local area. The purple color indicates that stagnant blood and fluids have been drawn up to the surface and out of the muscles and deeper tissues. Here at the superficial layer, the stagnation is more easily dispersed, by liniments, massage, poultices, and plasters. If there is no stagnation, the skin will get red while the cup is on, but the redness will quickly fade when the cup is removed.

It is easy to forget about the bruising until you see someone else's reaction to it. I have sometimes forgotten to warn people about the bruising. I remember treating a woman whose back went out the day before her wedding. I automatically cupped her back, and only then did I think to ask her what kind of dress she was wearing. It was, of course, backless. Although her back felt fine the next day, I gather the circular marks on her back caused some consternation during the ceremony.

Cupping and Frozen Shoulder

Cupping may also be used to treat more chronic injuries where there is impaired circulation or obstructed movement. One of my friends separated his shoulder slightly in a fall. The point of his shoulder hit the ground, pushing the end of the collarbone away from its attachment at the shoulder. Following some first-aid treatment and rest, it seemed to be healing fine, but after two weeks he could no longer raise his arm. I bled and then cupped around the point of the shoulder, and a gelatinous, clear substance was drawn out into the cup. He had ruptured the shoulder bursa. What I was removing was congealed fluids from the bursa sac. This jelly was gluing muscle fibers together, preventing normal movement and pressing on nerves, causing pain. Afterward he could immediately raise his arm. This was not the end of the treatment, but it was the turning point in his healing process.

CUPPING INDICATIONS
AND CONTRAINDICATIONS

While bleeding can be performed on almost any area on the torso except for the genitals, cupping is generally used on the surfaces of the body covered by large, thick muscles. The cups do not stick easily in bony areas like the wrist or ankles unless they are very swollen. Cupping *should not* be done

- over superficial veins or varicose veins.

- over areas of thin skin such as the face.

- over the eyes or ears, nose, or mouth.

- over the internal organs, such as the liver, stomach, and intestines.

- over open wounds or skin lesions, except insect bites, where it may be used to draw out the poison.

- on the back or abdomen of pregnant women.

- on people who bruise easily, people with lupus or hemophilia, or people who have skin sensitivity or circulation to the skin that is in any way impaired.

- (unless administered with extra care) on diabetics, children, and elderly people.

CLEANING YOUR CUPS

It is important to clean the cup after each use, particularly if cupping has been used in conjunction with bleeding. If used with bleeding, soak the cup(s) in bleach for thirty minutes and then wash thoroughly with soap and water. For cups with valves and a pump, set up the cup valve in a steel tray or pan with enough bleach to cover the area of the cup that actually made contact with the blood. Do not get water or bleach in the valve, as it can ruin the cup. Then set the cup in a pan of soap and water. It is important when using cups with valves to release the suction slowly so that blood does not spray up into the valve. Instead, it will touch

Cupping and Back Pain

Cupping can be very useful in treating low back pain and chronically tight upper back and shoulders. We know that an injury can rupture small blood vessels, causing blood to collect in the tissues. This blood congeals, disrupting the normal circulation of blood, qi, and fluids and preventing muscle fibers from sliding smoothly across one another. The disruption of normal circulation also interferes with the blood's function of nourishing muscles and tendons and makes the injured area susceptible to cold, both of which in turn cause further contraction or constriction. However, this can work both ways. Muscles that are chronically tight from stress, poor posture, or misuse can also restrict normal circulation and over time lead to stagnation of qi, blood, and fluids. This vicious circle, diagrammed here, is often the mechanism that perpetuates chronic back pain.

Injury
↓

Qi, blood, and fluids stagnate, blocking ——————→ Blood and fluids congeal; normal circulation   circulation of qi and blood is blocked

↑   ↓

Tight muscles constrict movement of qi, blood, and fluids   Muscles are not nourished; normal movement of muscle fibers is impeded

Tight muscles

Stress, poor posture, and overwork   Cold

Placing one or more cups on the tight areas of the back for 10–15 minutes or using a technique called "sliding cups" is often the first step in restoring normal circulation. To use sliding cups, cover the back with a thin layer of vegetable oil. Create suction in a cup and then slide it up and down the back. This method can be very effective, as it not only draws the stagnated fluids to the surface, but disperses them by pushing the circulation through the superficial tissues. After cupping, massage the back with a warming liniment such as U-I oil or Chinese massage oil (chapter 10). Cupping by itself can work wonders, but for chronic back pain it is generally used in conjunction with acupressure (chapter 13), moxibustion (chapter 16) if the back is cold and stiff, and proper exercise (chapters 5 and 6).

only the lip of the cup. *If you cup and bleed someone else, use plastic gloves to remove and clean the cups.* If you do cupping without bleeding, alcohol may be used instead of bleach, and the inside of the cups can be wiped with an alcohol swab or a cotton ball soaked in alcohol.

DISPOSING OF LANCETS

Lancets, like any medical waste product, should be disposed of properly. Sharp medical waste (sharps) can injure or infect sanitation workers if they are thrown in casually with other garbage. The rules for patients and pharmacy customers are different from those for medical professionals, who must have a licensed company dispose of medical waste. New York State law allows for household sharps to be disposed of with household trash, as long as they are in a puncture-resistant plastic container with a tight-fitting screw top. The container should be labeled "Contains Sharps." Other states or local laws may prohibit this. When you purchase lancets at a pharmacy, ask your pharmacist for instructions on how to dispose of them properly after use, or consult with your local public works department or trash collector.

CHAPTER 10

Liniments

The average Chinese pharmacy contains twenty or thirty different liniments, and there are probably hundreds available from various companies inside the United States and China alone. Many of these commercially available liniments are used to treat the muscle aches, bruises, contusions, and sprains associated with sports injuries. In the West, we tend to think of liniments as temporary palliatives, but the liniments used in Chinese sports medicine are powerful tools that can speed healing and reduce possible complications. Most liniments contain herbs that kill pain, but painkilling herbs are not mere analgesics that mask the pain. These herbs reduce pain by reducing swelling and inflammation, breaking up accumulations of blood and fluids, and restoring normal circulation to the injured area.

Over the years I have tried many different liniments on myself, on patients, on students, on fresh injuries, and on old injuries. Some of my colleagues and I even did comparison tests. We would try one liniment on a bruise or sprain on someone's arm and another on a similar injury on another part of the same person's body. I have found five liniments that are indispensable in treating sports injuries:

1. Trauma liniment.

2. Tendon lotion.

3. Chinese Massage Oil.

4. Black ghost oil.

5. U-I oil.

Liniments have certain inherent advantages over other methods of herbal substances applied to injured areas:

- They are easy to administer: simply rub them into the affected area. Their effectiveness increases when they are used in conjunction with massage techniques.

- Liniments last a long time. Once the herbs have been extracted into alcohol or mixed with aromatic oils, they do not go bad, particularly if stored in a cool place out of the sunlight.

- Liniments are easily stored in small bottles, making them convenient to transport to work, the gym, or an athletic event.

The main disadvantage of liniments is that they need to be applied frequently to be effective. This is because the volatile aromatic oils and alcohol used to extract the herbal ingredients, which aid penetration into skin and muscle tissue, tend to evaporate quickly. This disadvantage can be offset somewhat by using the liniment to create a simple poultice. To use liniments in this way:

1. Wrap rolled gauze or a clean cloth around the injured area. If the injury is to an area like the chest or front of the shoulder, place a gauze pad over the injury and tape down the edges.

2. Wet the bandage with the liniment so it soaks through the cloth or gauze to the skin.

3. Cover with an elastic bandage or more rolled gauze or gauze pads and leave on for several hours or overnight.

TRAUMA LINIMENT

Trauma liniment (die da jiu), whose name in Chinese literally means "hit-fall wine," is the number one remedy for bruises, contusions, sprains, and fractures. Every kung fu school uses a form of trauma liniment to deal with the injuries incurred in daily training. Bruises are usually shrugged off by most athletes as minor injuries that will heal themselves, but over the centuries kung fu practitioners noticed that large bruises or repeated bruising in one area sometimes created accumulations of stagnant qi and blood that could cause serious health problems years later. Trauma liniment was developed to disperse these accumulations and treat sports injuries, thereby prolonging an athlete's career and health.

Trauma liniment has so many uses that I keep gallons of it at my clinic and martial arts school. It is invaluable in treating the

Cautions

- Liniments are for external use only.

- Liniments and medicated plasters should not be used simultaneously. The ingredients in the plaster may interact with the liniment, causing burns or skin irritation. If you have been using a liniment, wash the area thoroughly and give the skin time to breathe before applying a plaster.

- Liniments should not be used in conjunction with direct heat such as a heating pad, wet heat, or hot shower (unless specified).

- Liniments should not be applied to mucous membranes such as the eyes, genitals, or mouth.

- Liniments should not be used on open wounds, cuts, or abrasions.

- Liniments should not be used on the lower abdomen of pregnant women.

wide variety of contusions, sprains, and strains so common to sports activities. Contusions of the shin are a common martial arts injury, where the effectiveness of trauma liniment is unanimously appreciated. Kicks to the shin or accidental shin-to-shin contact can be extremely painful, often causing the formation of large lumps on the shin. Rather than using ice to reduce swelling, massage trauma liniment into the contused area. Gently flatten the lumps, thereby dispersing the stagnant qi and blood. Reapply every few hours or soak cotton balls or gauze pads in the liniment and put them over the bruised area. Then cover with rolled gauze or an elastic bandage to hold the soaked material against the skin. Do not wrap too tightly. Often by the next day the lumps and much of the pain will have disappeared.

Although each kung fu school prides itself on having a unique formula that is superior to all others, most trauma liniments are fairly similar. All contain ingredients that stop pain, reduce swelling and inflammation, and disperse stagnant qi and blood. The following recipe makes a good-quality trauma liniment that is effective for treating a wide variety of sports injuries. In this formula, cooling and warming herbs are carefully balanced so that the cooling herbs reduce inflammation and swelling as effectively as ice, while the warming herbs kill pain, promote circulation, and break up accumulations of blood and fluids.

TRAUMA LINIMENT: EXTERNAL USE ONLY

12 grams	Da huang	*Rhizoma rhei* (rhubarb)
12 grams	Zhi zi	*Fructus gardenia jasminoidis* (gardenia)
12 grams	Hong hua	*Flos carthami tinctorii* (safflower)
12 grams	Huang bai	*Cortex phellodendri* (phellodendron bark)
12 grams	Mo yao	*Myrrha* (myrrh)
12 grams	Ru xiang	*Gummi olibanum* (frankincense)
12 grams	Xue jie	*Sanguis draconis* (dragon's blood)
12 grams	Lu lu tong	*Fructus liquidambaris taiwanianae*
12 grams	Dang gui wei	*Radix angelica sinensis* (tang kuei tails)

This recipe makes 1 gallon of trauma liniment. The herbs will have already been dried or otherwise prepared by the Chinese pharmacy or herb supplier. Simply put the herbs in a jar with 1 gallon of vodka or rice wine (80–100 proof).

Making Liniments with Alcohol

One of the easiest ways to extract the herbal ingredients into a liquid is to soak them in alcohol. Both trauma liniment and tendon lotion are made this way. One might think that the greater the strength of the alcohol, the stronger the liniment will be, but in fact vodka or a strong rice wine work far better than grain alcohol. Vodka and rice wine are roughly 50 percent alcohol and 50 percent water. Both alcohol and water are needed to maximize extraction of the herbal ingredients. Place the herbs in a glass jar and add 1 gallon of vodka or rice wine. Do not use a plastic container. Use a jar with a cork or a top that will seal firmly. Screw-on tops should be taped shut to create a better seal. If you buy the herbs and don't get around to making the liniment right away, it is okay—the herbs will keep for nine months to 1 year if they are stored in a plastic bag.

Store the jar out of the light and away from radiators or heaters. Shake the jar as often as you can. Every day is best, although I have forgotten for months at a time and the liniment came out fine. Six weeks is the minimum time for the herbs to soak before using the liniment, but a year or more is better. If you can't wait, after 6 weeks pour a little off the top into a small glass bottle for immediate use and store the rest. Liniments that are extracted with alcohol never go bad, and as the recipes in this book will make a gallon of liniment, there will be more than enough to treat several injuries. For daily use it is best to pour the liniment into smaller bottles that can be easily transported or stored in a first-aid kit, cabinet, or drawer. Plastic is not recommended for long-term storage, although when traveling, I have stored liniments in plastic bottles for as long as a month without a problem.

How to Apply Trauma Liniment

1. **Bruises:** Put a small amount of trauma liniment in your palm and pat it gently into the injured area. This helps it penetrate. Then use your thumb or three fingers to massage sore spots and break up lumps or accumulations. Start lightly and gradually work the liniment in deeper as the pain subsides.

2. **Muscle pulls:** Massage the liniment into knots in the muscle. Try to break up knots by following the direction of the muscle fibers (longitudinally). Also massage the liniment into the muscle attachments. For example, for a pulled hamstring:

   • Pat the liniment into the painful area.

   • Then use the thumb or three fingers to massage in circles around the sore area.

   • Use the thumb to break up knots by massaging upward toward the head and downward toward the feet, following the direction of the muscle fibers.

   • Finally, massage the liniment deep into the crease below the buttocks and the area behind the knee, as the hamstrings have tendon attachments to bone in both these areas.

3. **Sprains and strains:**

   • Massage trauma liniment gently into the injured area. If there is swelling, put some liniment on the tip of your thumb or fingertips. Start at the edge of the swelling and rub in small circles around the edge with your thumb or fingertips.

   • Add a little more of the liniment to your fingertips and lighten your pressure as you move inward, slowly and gently working the liniment into the center of the swollen area.

- Apply more liniment to your fingertips and direct your circles outward from the center, gently pushing stagnant fluids and blood away from the swollen area so they can be reabsorbed.

TENDON LOTION

While trauma liniment is ideal for bruising and acute, inflamed, and swollen injuries, tendon lotion is used for chronic injuries to tendons and ligaments. These kinds of injuries run the gamut from old sprains that are slow to heal to recurring tendonitis. While trauma liniment contains a balanced mix of cooling and warming herbs that do not overheat an inflamed area, tendon lotion contains many more warming herbs that act to stimulate local circulation. The inclusion of these warming herbs is very important in treating chronic tendon injuries like tennis elbow because, unlike muscles, tendons do not have an extensive direct supply of blood. That is why these kinds of injuries can be recalcitrant and slow to heal. Increasing local circulation also prevents cold and dampness from penetrating the injured area.

Tendon lotion should not be used when there is residual inflammation. In cases of tendonitis, it is not uncommon for there to be residual inflammation, which can flare up if direct heat or warming liniments, poultices, and plasters are applied. So how do you know if there is residual inflammation? If heat makes your injury feel better, it is probably safe to use tendon lotion. If you are still not sure, apply tendon lotion twice a day for 1 or 2 days. If the pain worsens, switch to trauma liniment.

TENDON LOTION: EXTERNAL USE ONLY

12 grams	Cao wu	*Radix aconiti kusnezoffii* (wild aconite)
12 grams	Chuan wu	*Radix aconiti carmichaeli* (Sichuan aconite)
12 grams	Tao ren	*Semen persica* (peach kernel)
12 grams	Ma huang	*Herba ephedrae* (ephedra)
12 grams	Zi ran tong	*Pyritium* (pyrite)

12 grams	Mo yao	*Myrrha* (myrrh)
12 grams	Ru xiang	*Gummi olibanum* (frankincense)
12 grams	Da huang	*Rhizoma rhei* (rhubarb)
12 grams	Lu lu tong	*Fructus liquidambaris taiwanianae*
12 grams	Zhang mu	*Lignum camphora* (camphor wood)

The herbs in tendon lotion are extracted with alcohol. This recipe makes 1 gallon of trauma liniment. The herbs will have already been dried or otherwise prepared by the Chinese pharmacy or herb supplier. Simply put the herbs in a jar with 1 gallon of vodka or rice wine (80–100 proof).

How to Apply Tendon Lotion

Put a small amount of tendon lotion on the ball of your thumb or on the pads of two or three fingers. Massage the liniment gently into the injured area. Pressure should be deep enough to penetrate, but not so deep as to be painful. Make small circles with your thumb or fingers to work the liniment into the injured tissues. Continue to rub the liniment into the area for several minutes, adding more to your fingers as needed. For an injury like shin

Frankincense and Myrrh

Frankincense (ru xiang) and myrrh (mo yao) are both tree resins. Long ago, traders from the Middle East traveled the Silk Road to bring these herbs to China. In the West, frankincense and myrrh have been used for embalming, as incense, or as ingredients in cosmetics, fragrant oils, and perfumes. In China, they became prized for their effectiveness in healing injuries and wounds. These two herbs often appear together in herb formulas because they act synergistically to kill pain, crack blood stagnation, and regenerate the flesh in cases of nonhealing wounds. Xue jie (dragon's blood) is a reddish tree resin similar to frankincense and myrrh. It is also included in many injury formulas. Xue jie was used in Europe in the sixteenth and seventeenth centuries to reduce the pain of gout.

splints, where small microtears in the muscle are pulling the muscle away from the bone, massage in circles gently toward the bone, using tendon lotion.

One patient with chronic tennis elbow had tried ice, physical therapy, and anti-inflammatories, to no avail. He came for one acupuncture session and then used tendon lotion every day, massaging it into his elbow with a vibrating acupoint massager he had ordered from a catalog. After the first treatment he never came back. Months later, he called to order more tendon lotion and to tell me he hadn't come back because his elbow was almost completely pain-free.

U-I OIL

U-I (pronounced "ooh-eee") oil is a blend of light aromatic oils. It is available as a patent remedy in most Chinese pharmacies. U-I oil contains cinnamon, peppermint, and lilac oils, as well as the tree resin xue jie (dragon's blood), an herb noted for its ability to relieve pain and dispel congealed blood. The main ingredient of U-I oil, however, is ai ye oil. Ai ye is known in the West as *Folium artemisiae,* or mugwort. In China, cigars made of mugwort leaves called "moxa sticks" are held close to the skin to heat up acupuncture points. This technique is known as "moxibustion" (see chapter 16). The natural oils found in the mugwort leaf have been extracted into U-I oil. These oils penetrate obstructions in the meridians, activate local circulation, and drive out cold, properties that make U-I oil useful in a variety of situations. Massage U-I oil into muscles and joints that ache in cold, damp weather. U-I oil can be used safely with wet heat in the form of hydrocollator packs or hot towels. Wet heat helps the oil to penetrate more deeply. U-I oil comes in a small glass bottle packaged inside a slender can. You may need more than 1 bottle if you are using it to treat chronic injuries or spreading it over large areas of the body.

- Massage U-I oil into muscles that are stiff and sore from overexertion.

- Massage U-I oil into stiff, cold muscles before exercising, to help them warm up or prepare them for stretching exercises.

- U-I oil can be massaged into areas that have been cupped (chapter 9) to help disperse stagnant blood and fluids that have been drawn up to the superficial layers of tissue.

CHINESE MASSAGE OIL

Chinese Massage Oil is made by the Oriental Herb Company in Chicago, Illinois (see appendix 2). It is an excellent liniment to massage into stiff, sore muscles because it penetrates deep muscle layers to promote the circulation of qi and blood. Chinese Massage Oil can also be used before hard physical training to warm up and prepare the muscles for exertion, thereby preventing pulled muscles. It can also be used after exercising or sports events to soothe sore muscles and relax tight areas. Before exercise, massage the oil into tight muscles, starting with long stroking movements and progressing to deeper kneading movements. Afterward, reapply the oil and let it penetrate for 10–15 minutes as the body cools down, before showering. Chinese Massage Oil can also be used

U-I Oil for Cold, Stiff Muscles

I frequently use U-I oil in conjunction with heat for back pain that worsens with cold, damp weather. It is not uncommon for this condition to affect people who do physical labor or exercise outdoors in inclement weather. Sweating or wearing sweaty clothes in cold, damp weather allows cold to penetrate muscles and joints, creating obstruction and pain. To help remove the obstruction and reduce pain, soak gauze or a paper towel with U-I oil. Place it over the painful area and cover with plastic wrap. Put a hot-water bottle, hydroculator pack, or hot wet towels on top and let the heat drive the oil into the muscles.

This technique also works very well for stiff necks due to drafts or air-conditioning blowing on the upper back and neck. This is a common problem in the summer when people are sweating and sit in front of the air conditioner or sleep with a fan or air conditioner blowing on them.

prior to performing flexibility and stretching exercises. Warming up the muscles in this way can enhance the effect of the exercises. As with all liniments, keep the oil away from the eyes and the genitals. Wash your hands after applying the oil so you don't accidentally rub your eye and irritate it.

One of my students experienced knee pain when he exercised or climbed the stairs. His lower back and hamstrings were very tight and inflexible. This prevented him from using his leg muscles properly, causing the knee joint to take the strain. I had him use Chinese Massage Oil in conjunction with flexibility exercises such as Knee Rotation and Phoenix Stretch—exercises 10 and 11 of the Daily Dozen (chapter 5). His knee pain disappeared within a few weeks.

BLACK GHOST OIL

Black ghost oil (hei gui you) is also called "hak kwai pain-relieving lotion." It is indispensable for bruises that are felt but not seen. Usually, these kinds of bruises occur in areas where there are thick muscles overlaying the bones. The deep layers of muscle tissue just above the bone are bruised and painful, but there is no visible swelling or discoloration at the surface. For this kind of deep bone bruise, black ghost oil is more effective than trauma liniment because it contains aromatic herbs and oils that are said to penetrate obstruction. These substances sink through the muscle tissue while dispersing blockages of qi and blood. Although black ghost oil sounds similar to Chinese Massage Oil, it penetrates more deeply, to strongly disperse obstructions, so it should be used sparingly and for this specific purpose only. Black ghost oil is available from almost every Chinese pharmacy. One bottle can easily treat several bone bruises.

SUMMARY

Trauma Liniment

FOR: Bruises, contusions, sprains, and strains where there is swelling and inflammation.

CONTAINS: Mix of cooling and warming herbs that relieve pain and reduce swelling and inflammation.

Tendon Lotion

FOR: Chronic injuries to tendons and ligaments such as repeated sprains or tendonitis.

CONTAINS: Warming herbs. Not for swollen, inflamed areas.

U-I Oil

FOR: Stiff, painful muscles and joints that are worse with the cold.

CONTAINS: Warming oils that activate the circulation and drive out the cold.

Chinese Massage Oil

FOR: Stiff, inflexible muscles. Penetrates deep into the muscles, improving local circulation. Use with flexibility exercises to help increase muscle pliability.

CONTAINS: Aromatic oils that penetrate muscles and increase local circulation.

Black Ghost Oil

FOR: Bruising that is felt but not seen.

CONTAINS: Aromatic oils that disperse blockages and strongly penetrate to the deep muscle layers just above the bone.

CHAPTER 11

Poultices and Plasters

Poultices and medicated plasters were once common remedies for muscle aches, torn muscles, and sprains. These therapies have all but gone out of fashion in the West, yet their effectiveness in treating sports injuries is unsurpassed. Thanks to China's martial traditions, a wide variety of poultices and plasters is still available today. Poultices and plasters are known collectively as *gao* in Chinese.

POULTICES

Poultices are generally composed of finely powdered herbs that are mixed with an aqueous or viscous medium. This combination produces a thick, mudlike paste that molds to the injured area and penetrates into the tissue. This paste is then covered with clear cloth and an elastic bandage to hold the mixture firmly against the skin. Different mediums may be chosen to enhance or modify the effect of the herbal powder. Common mediums for sports injuries are Vaseline, egg whites, green tea, or alcohol. Poultices tend to have a stronger effect than medicated plasters, and their therapeutic action can be adjusted by changing mediums. The main drawback to poultices is that they require preparation and they can be messy, particularly when used on areas that are difficult to wrap, such as the shoulder or thigh.

A wide variety of medicated plasters can be purchased at Chinese pharmacies. Medicated plasters consist of sheets or rolls of adhesive bandage with herbs and oils impregnated into the adhesive. Most are as easy to apply as a Band-Aid. Simply peel off the plastic backing and spread out over the injured area.

San Huang San: The Herbal Ice

Ice is about the only poultice still recommended by Western doctors and physical therapists. Many sports medicine books advocate putting ice packs on pulled muscles, sprains, and contusions. Unfortunately, ice has its drawbacks. As we saw in chapter 2, ice temporarily reduces inflammation, but it increases the stagnation of qi, blood, and fluids and causes contraction of muscles and sinews. These side effects ultimately retard the healing process and increase the potential for injury. The use of ice is so ingrained and unquestioningly accepted in our culture that many of my patients look at me as though I'm crazy when I suggest that ice may make matters worse. This is simply because they don't know there is an alternative.

Warrior monks and martial arts masters have known for centuries of a simple poultice that is remarkably effective for the injuries sustained during hard physical training. San huang san (three yellow powder) is composed of three cooling herbs that reduce inflammation while dispersing congealed blood and fluids. San huang san is probably the single most useful herbal formula for the first-aid treatment of sprains, strains, muscle pulls, or severe contusions. San huang san can even be used for a simple closed fracture where the bone has not penetrated the skin. Where you would normally use ice for an acute injury, use san huang san instead. The following formula is a modified form of san huang san. Additional herbs have been added to enhance its effect.

SAN HUANG SAN: EXTERNAL USE ONLY

Da huang	*Rhizoma rhei* (rhubarb)
Huang qin	*Radix scutellaria baicalensis* (skullcap root)
Huang bai	*Cortex phellodendri* (phellodendron bark)
Pu gong ying	*Herba taraxaci mongolici* (dandelion)

| Zhi zi | *Fructus gardenia jasmonoidis* (gardenia) |
| Hong hua | *Flos carthami tinctorii* (safflower) |

The herbs will have already been dried or otherwise prepared by the Chinese pharmacy or herb supplier. Use equal amounts of each herb. Have the herbs ground to a fine powder. See appendix 2 for a list of Chinese herb stores that will perform this service. Ten grams of each herb will yield a fairly large bag of powder, good for several applications. It is a good idea to always have a supply of san huang san available in your first-aid kit, because when you need it you probably won't be near a store that sells Chinese herbs. The herbs will be mixed with a medium to make a poultice. It is possible to premix san huang san if you use a medium such as Vaseline.

Knee Injuries and San Huang San

San huang san mixed with egg whites is very effective for acute knee injuries. It reduces the swelling and inflammation more effectively than ice, allowing the athlete to more quickly regain range of motion in the knee joint. While you are waiting to see your doctor or to get an MRI, you can begin treatment right away by using san huang san.

One of my associates injured his knee tubing behind a motorboat. The next day, his knee was swollen, painful, and difficult to bend. We both suspected a torn meniscus, the cartilage lining the articular surface of the knee. The joint was too swollen to manipulate, so I had him apply a poultice of san huang san for 2 days. This reduced the swelling enough that he could bend and straighten his knee almost completely. I performed acupuncture and gently manipulated his leg. It slipped back into alignment with a soft click and he was able to walk almost normally. Another poultice of san huang san reduced the residual swelling. By the time he got the MRI, which confirmed that the injury was a meniscus tear, he was walking normally and already performing strengthening and flexibility exercises.

Making a Poultice with San Huang San

To make a poultice with san huang san, mix the powdered herbs with a medium until you have a thick paste the consistency of mud. You need enough of this paste to cover the injured area. Apply the paste thickly like cake frosting to the injury. Then cover with gauze pads or paper toweling, followed by a wrapping of rolled gauze. The gauze may be covered with an elastic bandage to press the paste firmly against the skin. The bandage should be firmly in place, but not so tight that it restricts the circulation. In general, tightly compressing a sprain or any injury that is swollen is not a good idea. It may reduce swelling temporarily in the injured area, but ultimately it will also reduce normal circulation and increase the stagnation of blood and fluids.

Severe Contusions

Severe contusions to muscles can be serious injuries, but conventional medicine has little to offer in the way of treatment. These injuries are usually caused by a fall or an impact to the belly of a large muscle or group of muscles like the quadriceps muscles of the thigh or the biceps. Muscle tissue is laced with a large number of blood vessels. The impact ruptures many small blood vessels, causing the muscle to fill with blood and swell. This type of injury can be extremely painful. Usually, severe contusions are treated with RICE (rest, ice, compression, and elevation) and painkillers. It is believed that the blood will gradually be absorbed by the tissues and that the ruptured capillaries will slowly heal on their own. In fact, in many cases pain and restricted movement remain for years afterward.

In Chinese medicine, severe contusions are considered to be serious injuries that need immediate and correct treatment. Blood that stagnates in muscle tissue does not necessarily reabsorb. It can congeal and harden, gluing muscle fibers together and blocking normal circulation in the local area. This in turn creates pain and stiffness that does not always abate with time. Such injuries are often exacerbated by the application of ice, which further constricts tissue and congeals the blood.

Areas like the hamstring muscles or the shoulder can be very difficult to wrap. For these areas, apply a thinner layer of san huang san, almost as if you are painting on the mixture. Then cover with gauze squares and tape down the edges or, on a large area like the hamstrings, use rolled gauze to cover the area.

Several mediums may be used for making poultices:

1. **Vaseline:** Vaseline is a good all-purpose medium. Melt the Vaseline and mix it with the powdered san huang san. As the mixture cools, it congeals into a thick, gooey paste. At my clinic, we premix san huang san with Vaseline and store it in a jar out of the sunlight so it is ready to use.

Blockages caused by severe contusions create a drain on the body's energy. The body must now work harder to circulate blood and qi through this restricted area. It is believed that blockages of this kind can eventually affect the internal organs via the meridian system, leading to internal problems that manifest only years later.

San huang san is the key first-aid treatment for severe contusions. I often use san huang san in conjunction with trauma pills (chapter 15) to address the problem from the interior and exterior simultaneously. For instance, one of my students was struck hard in the bicep during a martial arts class. His whole arm from shoulder to elbow became swollen and turned a lurid black and blue. I applied san huang san mixed with egg whites and had him take a trauma pill. The next day the swelling was down and the bruising had started to fade. Within a week his arm looked normal again. I have had similar experiences with a volleyball player who severely bruised the inside of her forearms and a pushcart vendor who fell against a steel step. His whole thigh was massively swollen with blood. The doctors did nothing. A few days of trauma pills and san huang san mixed with egg whites and the injury began to heal. A week later his leg was fine. Contrast these experiences with a woman who fell on her lower leg, rupturing blood vessels in the calf and shin area. Except for painkillers and ice, it went untreated. A year later it was still discolored, painful, and sensitive to the cold.

2. **Green tea:** Green tea has a somewhat cooling effect on the body, so as a medium it can enhance the anti-inflammatory, cooling effect of san huang san. Simply make a cup of green tea and mix the tea with the powdered san huang san.

3. **Egg whites:** Egg whites are used as a medium when the injury is to the muscle and tendons and the cartilage. Not only do egg whites direct the action of the formula to these structures, but traditionally egg whites themselves have been used to treat sprains and strains. I know several Italian Americans who learned this trick from their grandmothers. For suspected or confirmed meniscus tears, sprains, pulled or torn muscles, or severe contusions to muscle tissue, mix san huang san with egg whites to make a paste.

Sinew-Bone Poultice

This poultice is used primarily for chronic (stage 3) sinew injuries (see chapter 3). It is ideal for sprains or bone fractures, where the swelling and inflammation are gone but residual pain and stiffness remain. The sinew-bone poultice can also promote healing of overstretched ligaments, a common complication of wrist and ankle sprains. Unlike san huang san, which contains many cooling, anti-inflammatory herbs, the sinew-bone poultice is composed of many warming ingredients aimed at strongly stimulating circulation to damaged tissues. It should be used only after all signs of inflammation are gone. It is particularly useful if the joint is more painful in cold and damp weather.

SINEW-BONE POULTICE: EXTERNAL USE ONLY

3 grams	Chuan Wu	*Radix aconiti carmichaeli* (Sichuan aconite)
3 grams	Cao wu	*Radix aconiti kusnezoffi* (wild aconite)
15 grams	Bai zhi	*Radix angelicae dahurica*
6 grams	Mu xiang	*Radix aucklandia* (costus root)
9 grams	Hou po	*Cortex magnoliae officinalis* (magnolia bark)

9 grams	Xiao hui xiang	*Fructus poeniculi vulgaris* (fennel)
9 grams	Rou gui	*Cortex cinnamomum cassia* (cinnamon bark)
15 grams	Ru xiang	*Gummi olibanum* (frankincense)
15 grams	Mo yao	*Myrrha* (myrrh)
15 grams	Xue jie	*Sanguis draconis* (dragon's blood)
15 grams	Qiang huao	*Rhizoma et Radix notoptergii*
15 grams	Duhuo	*Radix angelica pubescentis*
15 grams	Xiang fu	*Rhizoma cyperi rotundi* (cyperus tuber)
15 grams	Niu xi	*Radix achyranthis bidentatae*
15 grams	Xu duan	*Radix dipsacus* (teasel root)
15 grams	Zi ran tong	*Pyritium* (pyrite)
15 grams	Mu gua	*Fructus chaenomelis*
15 grams	Hu gu	*Os tigris* (tiger bone)*
24 grams	Dang gui	*Radix angelicae sinensis* (tang kuei)
24 grams	Zi jing pi	*Cortex cercis chinensis* (rosebud bark)

The herbs will have already been dried or otherwise prepared by the Chinese pharmacy or herb supplier. Have the herbs ground to a fine powder. Melt Vaseline and mix with the powdered herbs to make a paste. Using Vaseline is particularly ideal if you want to pre-mix the formula. Alternatively, mix the powder with vodka, whiskey, or rice wine and cook it, stirring occasionally, until the alcohol burns off and a thick, mudlike paste is left. Cooking with alcohol increases the circulation-enhancing, warming effect of the poultice. It is particularly useful if discomfort is exacerbated by cold.

Caution: This poultice should be used only on the limbs, for fractures or chronic sprains. It should not be applied to the head or over the internal organs.

---

* The traditional recipe calls for tiger bone. As tigers are an endangered species, this herb is generally replaced with dog or cat bone. Many modern herbalists simply leave out this ingredient altogether and feel that its absence does not diminish the efficacy of the formula.

*   *   *

Once the paste is made, apply this poultice in the same fashion as san huang san. The sinew-bone poultice can be left on for up to 24 hours. I usually recommend applying the sinew-bone poultice for 24 hours on and then 24 hours off for several days. This allows the skin to breathe. For overstretched ligaments, apply the poultice in this way for up to 2 weeks. Many people, myself included, cannot go to work with a poultice on their wrist or ankle. If this is the case, apply the poultice at night only and let the skin breathe during the day.

PLASTERS

Most of my patients prefer medicated plaster to poultices, because they are less messy, are easy to apply, and can be carried anywhere. Because many plasters contain camphor or menthol, you can feel the herbs penetrate the skin immediately, spreading warmth and relaxation to the injured area. Plasters do have a tendency to dry out and irritate the skin with repeated applications, so having them on for a day and off for a day can prevent burns and skin out-

Poultice, Plasters, and Sensitive Skin

Some people have sensitive skin. Poultices and plasters, particularly those that contain warming herbs, can irritate the skin, causing an itch or a rash. This happens most commonly with the sinew-bone poultice, gou pi plaster, and hua tuo anticontusion rheumatism plaster. Fair-skinned people seem particularly susceptible to this. If you do get a rash, simply remove the plaster or poultice and air out the skin. Never use poultices and plasters together with heating pads or other heat sources. This combination can overheat the area and cause a burn. If you have just had a heating pad on the injured area or just been in a sauna or Jacuzzi, let the skin cool before applying a poultice or plaster.

breaks. If a plaster becomes too hot, remove it immediately. You may have selected a plaster that is too warming.

One problem with plasters is that after being stored for a time, they lose some of their adhesive quality. Plasters that come as long rolls, packaged in a can, tend to retain their adhesive and aromatic properties longer. They have an additional advantage in that they can be cut to size or can cover large areas. If the plaster won't stick, place it face-up in a frying pan on low heat for several minutes or microwave it for 20–30 seconds to resoften the adhesive. If you are not near a stove or microwave, a hot radiator or other heat source can be used instead. The unused portions of the can-packaged plasters can be wrapped in plastic wrap and stored in the can. The smaller rectangular plasters that are packaged in cardboard should be placed in a sealed plastic bag and stored out of the sunlight once they have been opened.

Wu Yang Pain-Relieving Plaster

The package maintains that this plaster provides cooling pain relief. Although this plaster does not necessarily feel cool when it is on, it does contain cooling herbs. It is in many ways similar to san huang san, although it does not penetrate as deeply into the skin. It can be used in any situation where you might use san huang san—sprains, strains, and torn or pulled muscles where there is swelling, heat, and inflammation. This pain-relieving plaster can be very useful for chronic tendonitis that is exacerbated by heat. Wu Yang pain-relieving plasters come packaged in cans or in boxes.

Yunnan Paiyao Plaster

Yunnan paiyao was mentioned in chapter 8 because of its effectiveness in stopping bleeding and healing wounds. Yunnan paiyao plasters take advantage of another property of yunnan paiyao, its ability to move stagnant blood. Because yunnan paiyao is relatively neutral in temperature, these plasters can be used for acute injuries, even if there is swelling or inflammation. Perhaps the best all-around plaster for traumatic injury, yunnan paiyao plasters are particularly useful for acute sprains with accumulations of blood and fluids.

701 Plaster

This is a slightly warming plaster. The 701 plaster contains many herbs that reduce pain by breaking up accumulations of qi and blood. These are combined with herbs that help heal damaged muscles, tendons, and ligaments. This plaster is stronger and more warming than the previous two plasters. It should not be used while inflammation, heat, and redness remain. One simple guideline is, if heat increases the pain, use the yunnan paiyao plaster or the Wu Yang pain-relieving plaster.

Doctors in China use 701 plaster to treat bone spurs. I have found it to be remarkably effective for bone spurs in areas that are not covered by thick muscle—heel spurs or bone spurs in the shoulder.

Hua Tuo Anticontusion Rheumatism Plaster

This is a still more warming plaster suitable for stage 3 sinew injuries (3–4 weeks after the initial injury), when there is still residual stiffness and pain. Hua tuo plasters are particularly useful when there is impaired circulation that has allowed cold to penetrate the injured area. If the area is cold to the touch or sensitive to the cold, this plaster is probably the correct choice. Hua tuo plasters are also good for chronic injuries that ache in cold, damp weather.

Gou Pi Plaster

The gou pi plaster (kou pi plaster) is the strongest of the plasters that can be bought in a Chinese pharmacy. In the other plasters described, the herbs are impregnated into the adhesive. In gou pi plasters, the herbs have been mixed with pine resin. Pine resin helps the other herbs to penetrate deeply through muscle tissue, down to the level of the bone.

The gou pi plaster consists of a piece of leather folded in half. When you pull the halves apart, you will see something that looks like a glob of hardened tar. This glob is the herbal mixture already cooked into a pine resin base and allowed to dry. Heat the plaster in a toaster oven or microwave or face-up in a frying pan over a low flame. In a pinch, you can hold the plaster near a candle flame. Let the heat soften the pine resin. As it softens, you can open and refold the plaster several times to spread the mixture more evenly over the leather. Let the plaster cool a little and then apply. Gou pi plasters can be used 2 or 3 times. Simply reheat to soften the pine resin and reapply.

Gou pi plasters are particularly useful for injuries to tendons, ligaments, and bones. They are somewhat warming and should be used after the initial inflammation and swelling have been reduced. Gou pi plasters penetrate through and disperse accumulations of qi, blood, and fluid. They also strongly stimulate local circulation, which helps damaged tissues to heal more quickly.

SUMMARY

San Huang San

- Cooling.

- Use instead of ice for stage 1 sinew injuries with redness, swelling, and inflammation:

  – sprains.

Pine Resin

As you probably know from climbing pine trees as a child, pine resin is extremely sticky and hard to remove. Pine resin will stain clothes, and some residue will probably remain on the skin after you remove the plaster. Mineral spirits can help to remove this residue. Shave off any hair in the injured area before applying a gou pi plaster. The pine resin will adhere to the hair, making the plaster almost impossible to remove. The first time I put a gou pi plaster on my sprained wrist, I could not get it off the next day. It took a combination of pulling and tugging and snipping hairs with scissors to remove it. Now I remember to remove any hair from the area to which I am applying the gou pi plaster.

- strains.

- pulled muscles.

- Primary treatment for severe contusions to muscles.

- Closed fractures.

Sinew-Bone Poultice

- Warming.

- Apply to stage 3 sinew injury or closed fracture.

- Use after initial swelling and inflammation are gone.

- Helps heal overstretched tendons and ligaments—cook with honey and alcohol.

Wu Yang Pain-Relieving Plaster

- Cooling.

- Similar to san huang san—can be used as a substitute.

Yunnan Paiyao Plaster

- Use on stage 1 or 2 sinew injuries or closed fractures.

- Breaks up accumulations of stagnant blood.

701 Plaster

- Warming.

- Reduces pain; breaks up accumulations.

- Use after initial inflammation and swelling are gone.

- Helps heal bone spurs.

Huo Tuo Anticontusion Rheumatism Plaster

- Warming.

- Helps heal injured areas that feel cold or worse with cold.

- Use on chronic injuries.

Gou Pi Plaster

- Warming.

- Strongly penetrates obstructions of qi, blood, and fluids.

- Treats closed fractures and sprains.

CHAPTER 12

Herbal Soaks

If you enter the clinic of a traditional bonesetter or martial arts physician, you might see a patient chatting with the doctor, his or her hand or foot immersed in a pot of herbs. Herbal soaks are a form of hydrotherapy used for centuries by practitioners of Chinese medicine. Because herbal soaks direct a penetrating heat into the body's tissues, they cannot be used for acute, swollen, or inflamed injuries. On the other hand, they are invaluable in treating injuries to the soft tissue where tension and spasm are restricting normal movement. This is a common problem in cases of severe sprains.

Herbal soaks are used primarily to treat hand, foot, ankle, and wrist injuries, because these body parts are easily immersed in a pot of liquid. Soaks can be used on larger areas of the body, such as the back, knee, or shoulder, by soaking towels in the herbal mixture and applying them directly to injured tissues.

Remember: Soaks *are not* used to treat bone fractures, because they have a dispersing, spreading effect on the qi and blood. Herbal formulas that treat broken bones (chapter 4 and chapter 16) are composed of herbs that break up stagnation while promoting the consolidation of qi and blood that is necessary for the bones to knit.

HOW TO MAKE AND USE HERBAL SOAKS

The two herbal recipes discussed in this chapter will get you 1 package of herbs when presented to a Chinese pharmacy or herbal supply company. Each package makes a soak that will last 7–10 days. Take 1 package of herbs. Put the herbs in a pot large enough to cover the injured area. Add about 2 gallons of water. There must be enough water to cover the injured area, so more water can be added if necessary. If the injury is to the foot or hand, add enough water so that the ankle or wrist will also be covered. Cover the pot and bring the liquid to a boil. Turn down the flame and simmer for 20–25 minutes. Then remove the pot from the stove.

At this point, the liquid is too hot to soak in. If the injury is to one of the extremities, you can bathe the injured area in the steam as the liquid cools. This warms the area and allows the steam to penetrate the superficial tissues. When the soak has cooled sufficiently—it is warm but not uncomfortably hot—soak the injured part for 15–20 minutes. By this point it will have cooled down quite a bit. If you are using towels, you can soak them in the liquid, let them cool briefly, and put them over the affected area.

Adding Vinegar and Alcohol

Vinegar and alcohol are often added to herbal soaks to enhance their therapeutic effect. Add a quart of rice wine or vinegar to the soak *after* you have simmered the herbs for 20–25 minutes and removed the pot from the stove.

VINEGAR: Softens spasms in the muscles and tendons and "smooths out" the flow of energy through the injured area.

ALCOHOL: Warms tissue and increases the local circulation by moving qi and blood through the blood vessels and meridians.

The towels will cool fairly quickly, so you will need several to keep a warm, penetrating heat on the injury for 15–20 minutes.

After using the soak, dry the skin and keep it warm and away from cold or drafts. Cover the pot. The soak can be used once or twice a day for up to 7 days. Simply reheat the liquid to a sufficiently warm temperature. There is no need to boil it again. As long as you keep the pot covered and reheat the soak every day, the liquid will not get moldly.

Some people like to strain out the herbs after the cooking procedure, but leaving them in the pot as you soak is easier and increases the strength of the herbal mixture.

TENDON-RELAXING SOAK

This is the most useful soak for the spasmed muscles and sinews that accompany muscle pulls and sprains. Use it after the initial inflammation is gone. A classic example of when to use the tendon-relaxing soak is that of a beach volleyball player who came to my office with a sprained ankle. It was a bad sprain with lots of swelling that restricted his ability to flex his ankle. Initially we applied san huang san to reduce the swelling and inflammation. By the second treatment, the swelling was down and the ankle looked almost normal, with only a slight residual swelling, but he could hardly bend it at all. I did acupuncture on the ankle, and then he soaked his foot and ankle in the tendon-relaxing soak twice a day for 2 weeks. After soaking, he performed range-of-motion exercises. He regained much of his mobility and was able to finish the season.

TENDON-RELAXING SOAK: EXTERNAL USE ONLY

15 grams	Dang gui wei	*Radix angelicae sinensis* (tang kuei tails)
15 grams	Hong hua	*Flos carthami tinctorii* (safflower)
15 grams	Su mu	*Lignum sappan* (sappan wood)
15 grams	Bai zhi	*Radix angelicae dahuricae* (anglica dahurica)
15 grams	Jiang huang	*Rhizoma curcumae longae* (tumeric rhizome)

15 grams	Wei ling xian	*Radix clemetidis chinensis* (Chinese clematis)
15 grams	Qiang huo	*Rhizoma et Radix notopterygii*
15 grams	Wu jia pi	*Cortex acanthopanacis radicis*
15 grams	Hai tong pi	*Cortex erythrinae variegatae*
15 grams	Niu xi	*Radix achyranthis bidentatae*
15 grams	Chuan lian zi	*Fructus meliae toosendan* (fruit of Sichuan pagoda tree)
15 grams	Tu fu ling	*Rhizoma smilacis glabrae* (glabrous greenbrier)
6 grams	Ru xiang	*Gummi olibanum* (frankincense)
9 grams	Chuan jiao	*Pericarpium zanthoxyli* (Sichuan pepper)
30 grams	Tou gu cao	*Herba speranskia tuberculata*

This formula constitutes 1 package of herbs, enough to make 1 soak that will last 7–10 days.

Bunions and Hammertoes

Bunions and hammertoes are two congenital problems that often end up being treated surgically. Both problems can be helped enormously by herbal soaks and massage. Bunions occur as the big toe begins to overlap the second toe. The metacarpal-phalangeal joint becomes inflamed and fluid accumulates. Eventually, calcification can occur, causing enlargement, stiffness, and deformation of the joint. Soaks and massage can soften the hardness and remove fluid accumulation, preventing the joint from calcifying. If caught early enough, it is possible to avoid surgical intervention.

Hammertoes are toes that are flexed downward into a curved or clawlike shape. For hammertoes, use the soak to relax the flexor tendons (on the undersides of the toes) that are contracted. Let the foot dry and air out for 10 ot 15 minutes and then massage tendon lotion (chapter 11) into the contracted tendons.

WARMING SOAK

This soak contains many warming herbs that strongly increase local circulation and drive cold and damp out of the injured tissue. Many of these warming herbs also reduce pain. This soak is much more warming than the tendon-relaxing soak and should be used only for stage 3 tendon injuries (chapter 3), where the muscle or the joint is stiff, painful, and sensitive to cold. Often the area is cold to the touch and pain worsens in cold, damp weather. Do not use this soak if there is any residual heat or inflammation in the area. When I was first studying Chinese medicine, I gave this soak to a friend who suffered from chronic back pain. She used towels to apply the soak to her back. It made the pain worse. Although it seemed like an old injury that needed warming up, in fact each time her back "went out" it became reinflamed and the tissues became sensitive to the hot temperature of the soak and the warming herbs. We discontinued the soak and used cooling liniments and plasters to alleviate the pain. If this soak makes the pain worse, it is usually because there is still residual inflammation. Discontinue and try more neutral or cooling liniments, poultices, or plasters.

WARMING SOAK: EXTERNAL USE ONLY

9 grams	Chuan wu	*Radix aconiti carmichaeli* (Sichuan aconite)
9 grams	Cao wu	*Radix aconiti kusnezoffii* (wild aconite)
9 grams	Chuan jiao	*Pericarpium zanthoxyli* (Sichuan pepper)
9 grams	Tou gu cao	*Herba speranskia tuberculata*
9 grams	Ai ye	*Folium artemisiae argyi* (mugwort leaf)
9 grams	Cang zhu	*Rhizoma atractylodis*
9 grams	Du huo	*Radix angelicae pubescentis*
9 grams	Gui zhi	*Ramulus cinnamomi* (cinnamon twig)
9 grams	Fang feng	*Radix ledebouriellae sesloidis*

9 grams	Hong hua	*Flos carthamii tinctorii* (safflower)
9 grams	Shen jin cao	*Herba lycopodii* (clubmoss)
9 grams	Liu ji nu	*Herba artemesiae anomalae* (artemisia)

This formula constitutes 1 package of herbs, enough to make 1 soak that will last 7–10 days.

SUMMARY

Tendon-Relaxing Soak

- Slightly warming.
- Relaxes muscles and tendons that are in spasm.
- Increases local circulation.
- Use for continued pain and restricted movement *after* the initial inflammation and swelling are gone.

My Ankle Injury

Several years ago, I injured an already weak ankle that had been sprained several times before. I was climbing on some boulders, and my foot landed on the point of a rock, pushing a bone out of place. The pain faded quickly, but over the next six months my ankle became stiff and weak. It would hurt, feel better for a week or two, and then become irritated again. I went to a colleague for acupuncture and realignment of the foot. Initially it felt only slightly better. We decided I should use the tendon-relaxing soak. I soaked the ankle twice a day for two weeks and regained full mobility, but it was sensitive to cold and occasionally sore. I switched to the warming soak for two weeks and the pain disappeared, allowing the ankle to slowly regain its strength.

Warming Soak

- Very warming.

- Treats stage 3 sinew injuries, where the area is painful and sensitive to cold or hurts more in cold weather.

- Relaxes tendons; warms and increases circulation to the local area.

CHAPTER 13

Sports Medicine Acupoints

One of the most common questions that people ask about Chinese medicine is, "How do acupuncture points work?" There is no simple answer to this question; however, modern science has conducted experiments and from these formulated several theories:

1. Stimulation of acupuncture points (or "acupoints") releases endorphins. Endorphins are peptides secreted in the brain that have a pain-relieving effect like morphine.

2. Acupuncture points somehow affect the nerves and can be used to block pain by preventing pain impulses from propagating from the spinal cord to the brain.

3. Research has indicated that the meridians conduct electrical currents and that skin resistance to these currents is less at acupoints. Acupoints may function like transformers or boosters by modulating the electrical activity in particular areas of the body.

While these theories are interesting, they do not fully explain the effects produced by stimulating acupoints with an acupuncture needle or massage techniques. In the past, much of the scientific research on acupoints was conducted to explain their effectiveness in managing pain. Such research was stimulated by the use of acupuncture analgesia as a replacement for general anesthetic during surgical procedures. Only recently has research been directed toward understanding the other effects acupuncture and acupressure produce in the body.

In Chinese medicine, acupoints are places where the flow of qi and blood can be influenced or modified to regulate the functional activities of the body. This means that acupoints can not only reduce pain, but also help regulate and harmonize the functions of the internal organs and the musculoskeletal system. In addition to the main meridians, which have deep connections to the internal organs, there are tendinomuscular meridians, which directly relate to the movement of muscles and joints. Through these meridians, acupoints can help relieve muscles that are in spasm and improve local circulation and joint mobility. This is why an acupoint like stomach 36 (ST 36) can be used by acupuncturists to treat a wide variety of problems:

- Gastrointestinal problems such as nausea, indigestion, bloating, and vomiting, because the stomach meridian has an internal connection with the stomach and intestines.

- Headache, hypertension, and dizziness, because the stomach meridian starts in the head and travels down to the feet. Therefore, ST 36 can be used to draw excess energy away from the head.

- Pain, injury, and weakness of the lower extremities, because the stomach meridian passes through the front of the hip, knee, and ankle.

In the West, we use a numbering system to list the acupoints on each meridian and diagram its pathway. In China, each point has a name, often poetic in nature. Sometimes, as in the case of ST 36 (zu san li), the name gives us insight into how the point is used. Zu san li means "leg three-li point" because of its ability to energize the legs so one could walk three more *li*, a distance of about three miles. The names of other points sometimes refer to their location or have more obscure meanings. I have included a standard translation of the Chinese name for each point, but only those names that give insight into the point's function will be discussed in detail.

So, will pressing ST 36 cure your torn meniscus? Probably not. However, stimulating acupoints is an important part of the first-aid treatment of sports injuries. Acupoints can help reduce pain and increase joint mobility, particularly if used in conjunction with the other therapies discussed in this book. They can also be used after the acute phase, during the healing and rehabilitation process, to direct the body's healing energies to the injured area. No one point will work all the time on every person, but the points discussed in this section are the strongest and work most of the time for most people. Acupoints can be used preventatively. If your legs ache after you run, don't ignore it until the pain becomes chronic. Remember, pain is a sign that energy and blood are not circulating freely. Use acupoints to relieve the pain and reestablish the free flow of qi and blood.

HOW TO STIMULATE ACUPOINTS

Acupoints can be stimulated with finger pressure. This is often just as effective as acupuncture. Direct pressure with the thumb, finger, or knuckles is one of the simplest and most effective methods of stimulating acupoints. Press the point lightly and shallowly, progressing slowly deeper until you feel a distending sensation around the point or a dull ache that spreads or travels outward from the point. Press and hold the point until pain subsides and you feel the muscles relax. In cases of fractures or suspected fractures, do not press acupoints that are directly over the site of the injury.

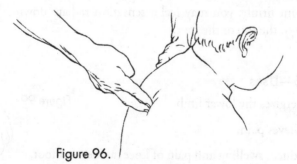

Figure 96.

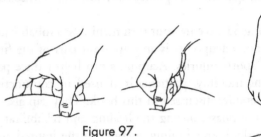

Figure 97.

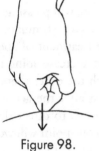

Figure 98.

THE LIMB ENERGIZERS

Stomach 36 (ST 36)   Zu san li (leg three-*li* point)
Large intestine 10 (LI 10) Shou san li (arm three-
                            li point)

These points energize the limbs by releasing energy into the meridians of the arms and legs. ST 36 is traditionally known as the "leg three-*li* point" because of its ability to energize the legs so one could walk three more *li*, a distance of about three miles. LI 10 is its corollary in the upper body, the "arm three-*li* point."

ST 36—Location

ST 36 is located about four fingers' width below the lower edge of the kneecap in the depression in the muscles outside the tibia (shinbone). (Figure 99.) If you press the point firmly, you may feel a sensation radiate down the leg to the top of the foot.

ST 36—Uses

- Energizes the lower limb.

Figure 99.

- Relieves pain.

- Reduces swelling and pain of knee, ankle, and foot.

LI 10—Location

LI 10 is located about two fingers' width below the elbow crease. (Figure 100.) If you turn the palm down and make a fist, it is just behind the muscle that stands out below the elbow.

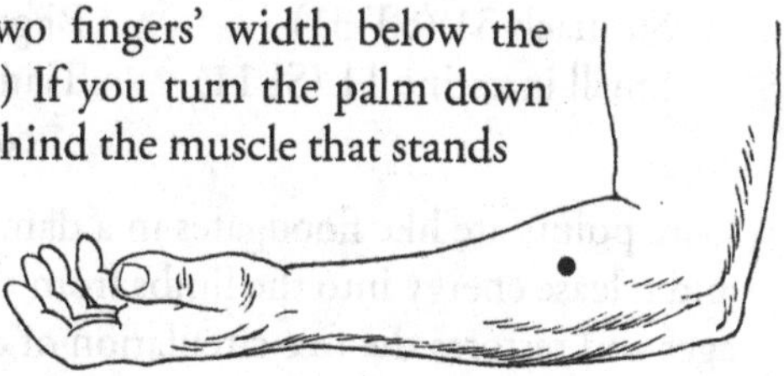

Figure 100.

LI 10—Uses

- Energizes the upper limb.
- Relieves pain.
- Reduces swelling and pain in the elbow, wrist, and hand.
- Reduces shoulder pain.

Acupoints Really Work

Teachers are often humbled by their students. I am always amazed by students who take an introductory class and then use what they learned, often achieving better results than experienced practitioners. Years ago, I taught a twelve-hour course in sports medicine. After completing the class, one of my students was at his gymnastics class when a fellow student sprained her ankle. He didn't have any liniments or poultices with him, but he remembered zu san li (ST 36). As he pressed the point, he watched the swelling literally shrink before his eyes. Acupuncturists learn many complex treatments and sophisticated techniques, yet often the most simple, direct treatments work the best. During the writing of this book, my left wrist and thumb began to ache from typing. I considered needling a number of acupuncture points on my wrist until I remembered my student's simple treatment. I pressed and held shou san li (LI 10). Within less than a minute the pain began to ebb away, reminding me not to underestimate even the simplest of treatments.

THE LIMB GATE POINTS

Stomach 31 (ST 31)	Bi guan (thigh gate)
Small intestine 11 (SI 11)	Tian zong (celestial constellation)

Gate points are like floodgates in a dam. They open the meridians and release energy into the limbs from the torso. This clears blockages and restores the free circulation of qi and blood.

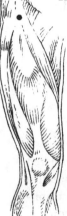

ST 31—Location

Trace a line from the pubic bone to the hip. The point is located in a depression just outside the sartorius muscle. (Figure 101.) This depression opens up when you bend the leg to sit cross-legged.

ST 31—Uses

• Releases energy from the torso into the leg.

• Alleviates pain in the thigh, hip, and leg.

• In conjunction with ST 36, energizes the lower limb.

• Stimulates to help prevent muscular atrophy of the leg (with ST 36).

Figure 101.

SI 11—Location

SI 11 is located in a depression in the center of the shoulder blade. (Figure 102.) This point is usually quite sensitive to pressure.

SI 11—Uses

• Releases energy from the torso to the arm.

Figure 102.

- Alleviates pain in the shoulder blade, arm, and elbow.

- Helps heal tendonitis of the elbow and wrist.

- Stimulates to help prevent muscular atrophy of the arm (with LI 10).

SHOULDER INJURY POINT

Triple heater 3 (TH 3)   Tian zong (central island)

TH 3—Location

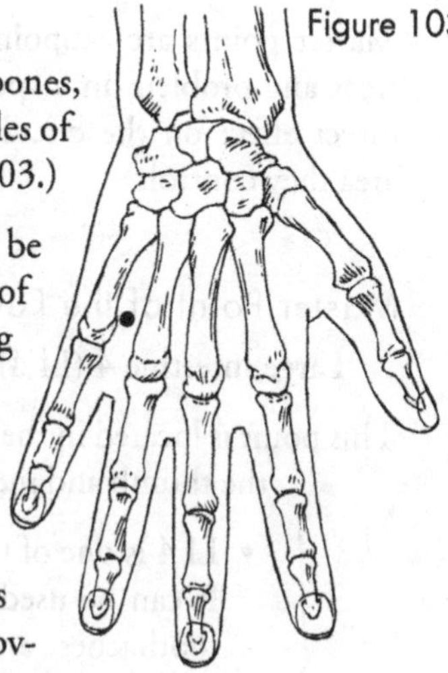

On the back of the hand, between the bones, in the depression just behind the knuckles of the ring finger and the pinkie. (Figure 103.)

Figure 103.

- Although SI 11 and LI 10 can also be used for shoulder injuries because of their energizing and energy-releasing effects, TH 3 is an effective point to treat shoulder pain and restricted movement in the shoulder.

- First press TH 3 on the same side as the injured shoulder. Then press TH 3 on the opposite side, while moving the shoulder in circles to increase range of motion. This works best if you can get someone else to press the point while you move your shoulder.

ANKLE INJURY POINT

Gallbladder 39 (GB 39)   Xuan zhong (suspended bell)

GB 39—Location

This point is located about three fingers' width above the lateral malleolus (the big bump on the outside of the ankle). (Figure 104.) Locate it in the depression between the bones of the fibula and tibia.

- The number one point for injuries to the ankle or the outside of the foot.

- This point relieves pain and opens the meridians that supply energy to the ankle and foot.

- GB 39 is a key point in treating ankle sprain and is particularly effective if used with ST 31 and ST 36.

MASTER POINTS

Master points are acupoints that can be used to treat any problem in a specific area. They have a direct effect on the circulation of energy in the area they control.

Figure 104.

Master Point of the Face and Head

Large intestine 4 (LI 4)   Hegu (connected valley)

This point is located in the center of the space between the thumb and index finger. (Figure 105.)

- LI 4 is one of the most versatile acupoints. It can be used for headaches, facial pain, toothaches, and pain in the front of the shoulder.

- Use with liver 3 (LIV 3), tai chiong (great thoroughfare) (Figure 106), to unblock all the meridians in the body and relieve pain and stagnation. This combination is also very effective for headaches.

  - *Do not apply heavy pressure to LI 4 if you are pregnant.*

Figure 105.

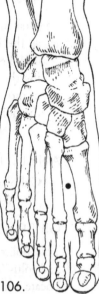

Figure 106.

Master Point of the Back

Bladder 40 (BL 40)   Wei zhiong
(bent middle)

This point is located on the center of the crease behind the knee. (Figure 107.)

- Press BL 40 to relieve any kind of back pain. For
  this purpose it is often used in conjunction with
  bladder 60 (BL 60), kun lun (kun lun mountains). (Figure 108.)

Figure 108.

Figure 107.

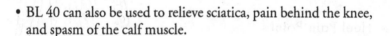

- BL 40 can also be used to relieve sciatica, pain behind the knee,
  and spasm of the calf muscle.

SPECIAL HAND ACUPOINTS FOR PAIN RELIEF

These are extra acupoints, not located on the main meridians, that
are particularly useful for restoring pain and mobility to injured
areas. Usually these points will be sensitive to pressure if there is
pain in the related area. In general, the point that is more sensitive
will be on the hand that is on the opposite side of the body from
the injury. For example, if the right side of the back is more
painful, the yao tong xue points on the left hand are more likely to
be painful. For several minutes, press and hold the point while
moving the injured area. The pain will often subside, and there
should be increased mobility.

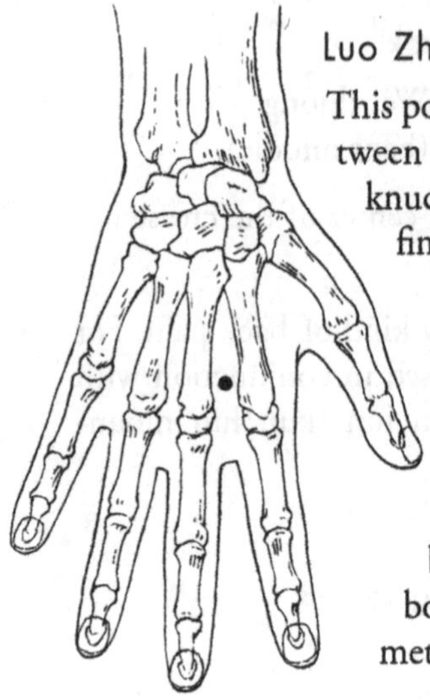

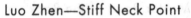

Luo Zhen—Stiff Neck Point

This point is located on the back of the hand, between the bones, in the depression behind the knuckles of the forefinger and the middle finger. (Figure 109.)

Yao Tong Xue—Lumbar Pain Points

There are two of these points, located on the back of the hand in the depression between the metacarpal bones, one between the metacarpal bones relating to the forefinger and middle finger and the other between the metacarpal bones relating to the ring and index finger. (Figure 110.)

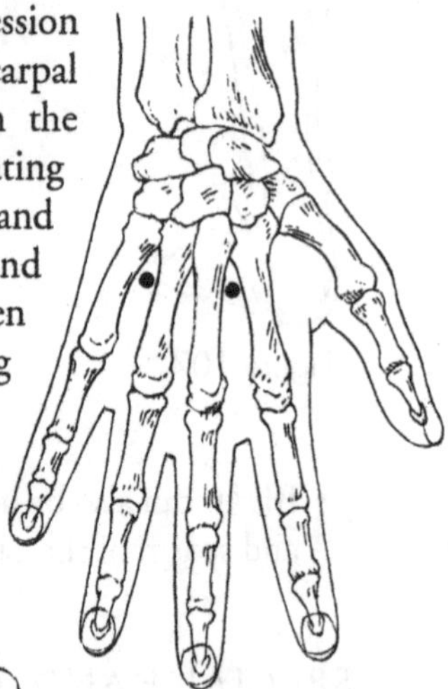

Figure 109.

Heel Pain Point

This point is located in the center of the heel of the palm, one finger's width above the wrist crease. (Figure 111.)

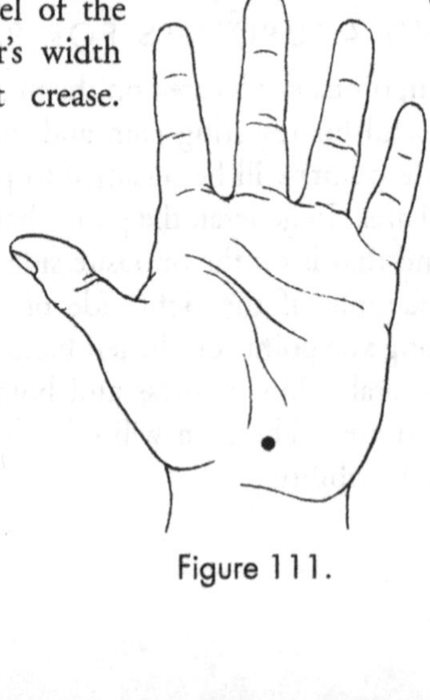

Figure 110.

Figure 111.

INFLUENTIAL POINT OF THE TENDONS AND LIGAMENTS

Gallbladder 34 (GB 34)   Yang ling quan
(yang mound spring)

GB 34—Location

This point is located in the depression just in front of and below the head of the fibula. (Figure 112.) The head of the fibula feels like a small knob of bone on the side of the leg a little below the knee. This point is slightly above and to the outside of ST 36.

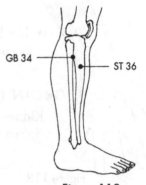

Figure 112.

GB 34—Uses

- Use to treat tendon ligament or cartilage injuries anywhere in the body.

- Particularly effective for tendon and ligament injuries to the knee, lower leg, and ankle.

- Use with GB 39 for ankle sprains.

- Combine with LIV3 to treat muscle spasms and cramps.

- GB 34 can be used with LIV3 to relieve the pain of fractured ribs.

RESPIRATION POINTS

Lung 5 (LU 5)   Chi ze (ulnar depression)
Lung 6 (LU 6)   Kong zui (gathering hole)

LU 5 and LU 6—Location

Lung 5 is in the elbow crease, just outside the tendon of the biceps. Lung 6 is in a depression on a line joining the base of the thumb to

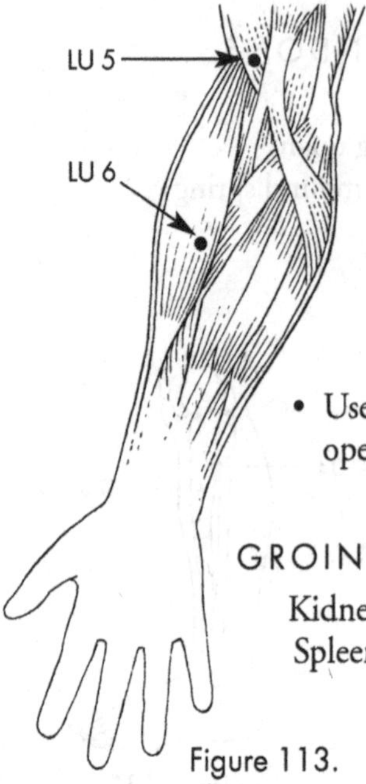

LU 5, about two-thirds the distance from the wrist crease to the elbow crease. (Figure 113.)

LU 5 and LU 6—Uses

• Press these points and gently pinch the bicep tendon for a person who is out of breath or feeling faint from overexertion.

• Use before an athletic event to stimulate and open up the lungs.

GROIN INJURY POINTS

Kidney 2 (KID 2)   Ran gu (blazing valley)
Spleen 4 (SP 4)   Gong sun (grandfather grandson)

Figure 113.

KID 2 and SP 4—Location

Both points lie in the groove between the muscles of the arch of the foot and the bones on the inside of the foot. (Figure 114.)

KID 2 and SP 4—Use

Press firmly with your fingertip or knuckle to relieve pain from a blow to the groin or testicles.

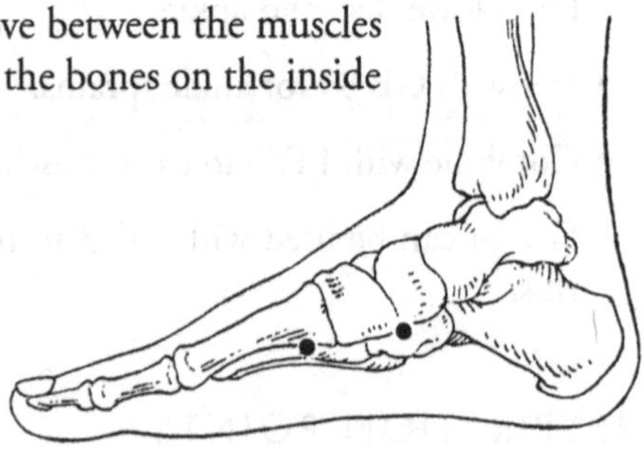

Figure 114.

NAUSEA POINT

Pericardium 6 (P 6)   Nei guan (inner pass)

P 6 is well-known for its ability to quickly relieve feelings of nausea; however, it is a powerful point with many uses.

P 6—Location

P 6 is located about two fingers' width above the wrist crease between the two prominent tendons in the center of the wrist. (Figure 115.)

P 6—Uses

- Nausea.

- Seasickness.

- Morning sickness.

- Stomachache.

- Stuffy feeling in the chest.

- Hangovers.

- Wrist pain/carpal tunnel pain (press gently).

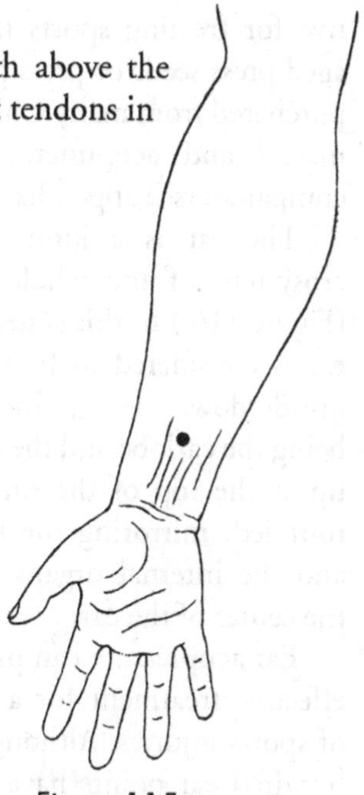

Figure 115.

EAR ACUPRESSURE

Ancient Chinese medical texts make mention of acupuncture points in the ear, but ear acupuncture and acupressure, as we know it today, did not develop until the mid–twentieth century. The acupoints of the ear were mapped by European physicians trained in acupuncture and Chinese medical researchers who combined their clinical observations with electrical measurements of the different parts of the ear. Today their findings are taught in every acupuncture school in the world.

Ear points are often stimulated with needles. However, clinical studies have shown that pressure with a small probe such as a matchstick, or the taping of small seeds or metal beads on the ear points, is equally effective. In fact, "seed pressure" is considered by many to be more effective than acupuncture because it can produce virtually continuous stimulation, and unlike acupuncture, this therapy does not require extensive training to use safely and ef-

fectively. This is the method I consider most effective for treating sports injuries. Prepackaged press seeds or press pellets can be
purchased from many Chinese pharmacies and acupuncture supply
companies (see appendix 2).

The ear is a kind of mi-
crosystem of the whole body.
(Figure 116.) In this system, the
ear is considered to be like an
upside-down fetus, the head
being the earlobe and the feet being
up at the top of the ear. The spine is
rounded, mirroring the fetal position,
and the internal organs are located in
the center of the ear.

Ear acupressure can provide safe and
effective treatment for a wide variety
of sports injuries. Although over one
hundred ear points have been cataloged and mapped, only a few key
points and concepts are needed to
treat most sports injuries. Ear
acupoints for the treatment of
sports injuries are divided into three categories:

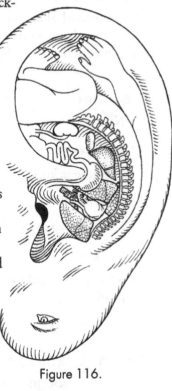

Figure 116.

Body Area

These are not so much points as areas of the ear that relate to areas
of the body. (Figure 117.) In general, their positions conform to
the microsystem idea of the upside-down fetus. Body area points
work best if you can find a specific point within the area that is
particularly sensitive to pressure. For example, for hip pain, look at
the hip area of the ear shown in the following ear chart. Probe the
hip area of one of your ears with the end of a matchstick or a small
probe to determine if one point within that area is more sensitive
to pressure than the others. If you cannot find a single point that is

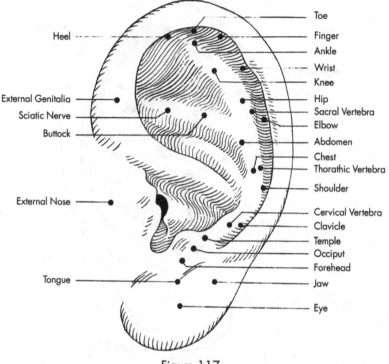

Figure 117.

sensitive, try the other ear. It is necessary to find only one sensitive point in one ear. This more sensitive point is the one that should be stimulated. If more than one area of the body has been injured (for instance, the hip and the knee), probe both of the corresponding areas of the ear to find a sensitive point in each area.

Specific Points That Relieve Pain and Calm the Spirit

Two points (Figure 118) are particularly useful for relieving pain and calming the spirit, which is easily agitated by pain and injury. These points are

- shen men—calms the spirit.
- sympathetic—calms the nerves.

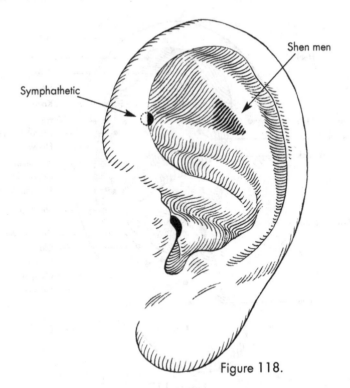

Figure 118.

Ear Points That Stimulate the Functioning of the Internal Organs

In chapter 2, I discussed the relationship between the internal organs and their associated issues. The healing of muscle, tendon, ligament, bone, and cartilage are dependent on the organs that supply them with fluids, blood, and nutrients. In Chinese sports medicine, three organs are considered to have direct connections with these tissues:

- Liver—tendon, ligament, cartilage.
- Spleen—flesh, muscles.
- Kidney—bones.

Like the body area points shown in figure 117, these "organ points" are not so much points as areas. Pick the point or points appropriate to the tissue that is injured. For a pulled muscle use the spleen point, for a sprained ankle the liver point, and for a bone bruise or broken bone use the kidney point. If a broken bone is accompanied by ligament damage, use both the liver and kidney points. If pulled muscles accompany a sprain, choose both the spleen and liver points. (Figure 119.)

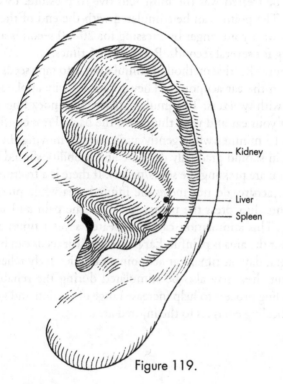

Figure 119.

STIMULATING EAR POINTS

A minimum of three ear acupoints will be stimulated:

1. the sensitive point corresponding to the body area injured.

2. shen men.

3. the sympathetic point.

To increase the effectiveness of the treatment, a fourth point that stimulates the organ associated with the injured tissue can be added:

4. spleen, liver, or kidney point(s).

These points need not be stimulated in both ears; one ear will suffice. Use the ear in which the point corresponding to the body area to be treated was the most sensitive to pressure. (See "Body Area.") The points can be stimulated with the end of the matchstick or with your finger by pressing for 20–30 seconds and then releasing for several seconds. Repeat 4 or 5 times.

A more effective method of stimulation is to tape seeds or press pellets on the ear acupoints. They are most easily applied and removed with tweezers. To stimulate, place your index finger on the front of your ear and your thumb on the back. Press continuously for 10–15 minutes while gently and carefully moving the injured area. Pain should gradually decrease and mobility should increase while you are pressing the seeds/pellets. If there is a fracture or suspected fracture, do not move the injured area while pressing the ear points. Just press the points to relieve the pain and stimulate healing. This stimulation can be repeated several times a day or whenever the area is painful. Ear pellets and ear seeds can be left on for several days at time. Ear acupoints can effectively relieve acute pain, but they may also be stimulated during the rehabilitation and healing process to help increase range of motion and guide the body's healing energies to the injured area.

CHAPTER 14

Massage for Sports Injuries

Traditional Chinese medicine includes very sophisticated massage methods that realign soft tissue and bone, energize the body, and treat internal disease. Being proficient in these methods usually requires study with an experienced practitioner of *tui na,* Chinese medical massage. However, incorporated within this more medically oriented massage system are techniques derived from folk medicine that have been practiced by ordinary people for generations. These techniques are effective, simple, and easy to learn. They can be used to treat your own injuries or to help family members or teammates.

Massage is an often underrated treatment modality that can be a very effective tool in the treatment of sports injuries. Massage, particularly when used in conjunction with liniments and soaks, can

- relieve pain.

- reduce swelling.

- relax muscle spasms.

- disperse accumulations of qi, blood, and fluids.

- stimulate circulation.

MASSAGE TECHNIQUES

There are six basic massage techniques you will need to treat most sports injuries.

Pressing

Pressing is used to direct pressure directly into the area to be stimulated. Pressing is particularly effective for stimulating acupoints (chapter 13) and can also be used to direct circulation of qi and blood to a particular area. Pressing can be performed with the palm, thumb, or one finger. Generally, the palm is more useful for large areas like the back, while the thumb and fingers can be used to press acupoints or to treat small areas like the wrist or ankle.

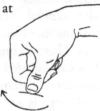

Figure 120.

Circular Pressing

Press slowly down into the flesh and muscle tissue until you reach the depth you wish to work at. Stay at that depth while making small circles with your thumb. For example, if the injury is to muscle, as in a pulled muscle, go down to the depth of the muscle and stay at that depth while making small circles with your thumb. This method is particularly good for dispersing local blockages of qi, blood, or fluids. It is very effective in the small areas around the bones and joints.

Figure 121.

Palm Pushing

Palm pushing is generally used on larger areas of the body, like the back or legs, that are covered by thick muscles. Press the palm slowly into the muscle tissue and then push the palm in long strokes along the muscles of the back or legs. Palm pushing relaxes

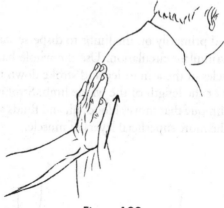

Figure 122.

the muscles and can be used to disperse stagnant qi, blood, and fluids or to direct circulation toward a particular area.

Pushing with the Thumb

This technique is the same as palm pushing, but the smaller surface area of the thumb makes it more suitable for working between muscles or in the smaller areas around joints and bones.

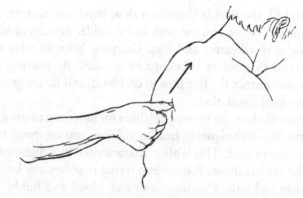

Figure 123.

Stroking

Stroking is used primarily on the limbs to disperse stagnation and swelling and stimulate circulation. Use the whole hand to gently grasp the muscles of the arm or leg and stroke down the length of those muscles or the length of the whole limb. Stroking is a more superficial technique that moves blood, qi, and fluids at the level of the skin and the more superficial layers of muscle.

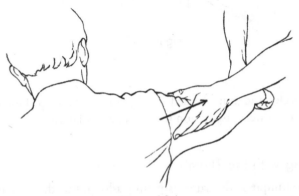

Figure 124.

Grasping

Grasp and lift the muscle tissue in a slow, rhythmic manner. This technique can be used on the neck and shoulder muscles as well as the muscles of the arms and legs. Grasping helps to relax tight muscles and to separate adhesions in muscles. By relaxing tight muscles that restrict the free flow of qi, blood, and fluids, grasping promotes local circulation.

In general, there are no set guidelines on how long to use a particular massage technique. In treating injuries, you are trying to get tight muscles to relax. This is often characterized by a slight softening in the muscle tissue. You are also trying to soften any knots in the muscle and reduce accumulations of blood and fluids. This may take anywhere from 30 seconds to 10 minutes depending on

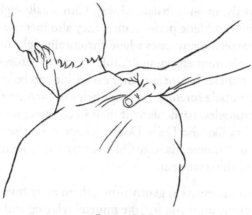

Figure 125.

the nature of the injury and where it is located. It is important for the technique to penetrate the tissues, but there should not be undue discomfort.

BRUISES

Bruises indicate that blood from ruptured blood vessels is trapped in the soft tissue. Although this blood often disperses on its own, sometimes it can congeal in the tissues, causing pain and soreness later. Massaging the area with trauma liniment (chapter 10) quickly disperses this stagnant blood and relieves pain and soreness.

- Put a small amount of trauma liniment in your palm and pat it gently into the injured area. This helps it penetrate.

- Then use your thumb or three fingers to massage sore spots and break up lumps or accumulations. Start lightly and gradually work the liniment in deeper as the pain subsides.

TIGHT AND SORE MUSCLES

Tight, sore muscles can simply be a result of playing too hard, but they can also indicate that you are overtraining or using the muscles improperly, in an imbalanced way. Chronically tight muscles not only hinder athletic performance, they also increase the risk of injury. I have seen many cases where chronically tight muscles discourage people from engaging in athletic activity altogether. Massaging sore muscles before and after exercising can be very helpful in reducing muscle soreness. Massage helps to increase the pliability of tight muscles, particularly if used in conjunction with flexibility exercises like the Daily Dozen (chapter 5). Use a liniment like U-I oil or Chinese Massage Oil (chapter 10) to increase the effectiveness of the treatment.

1. Grasp the muscles, gently lifting them away from the bone. Continue until you feel the muscles relaxing and softening.

2. Put some liniment onto the palm or thumb and use the palm or thumb to push along the length of the muscle. This pushes qi, blood, and fluids through the muscles and helps the liniment to penetrate. Repeat several times until the area is warm and there is a sense that circulation in the area has improved.

3. Circular push with the thumb into particularly tight areas. If there is a knot in the muscle, use the thumb to gently break up the knot.

4. Press any acupoint(s) that relate to the area of the body you are working on. For example, for the back use BL 40 and BL 60; for the arm use LI 10 (see chapter 13).

5. Finally, stroke down the muscle to further relax and warm tight areas. For example, if you are working on the arm, stroke from the shoulder to the elbow several times and then from the elbow to the wrist and fingers several times.

SPRAINS AND STRAINS

The treatment of sprains and strains is slightly more complex because there may be swelling as well as damage to tendons and ligaments.

If there is swelling:

1. Press gently around the edge of the swollen area.

2. Use *very* gentle circular pushing with the thumb to apply trauma liniment directly over the swollen area.

3. Circular push with the thumb around the edge of the swollen area, directing the force of the push outward.

4. Push outward from the swollen area with the thumb or palm. If the swelling is on the limb, in the knee area, for example, push from the knee toward the hip several times and then push from the knee toward the toes several times. This helps stagnant blood and fluids to be reabsorbed into normal circulation.

5. Press the acupoints that affect the injured area. For example, for the knee, use ST 31, ST 36, and GB 34.

If there is no swelling, as in a strain or chronic injury:

1. Repeat steps one through four of the massage protocol for sore, tight muscles.

2. Circular push with the thumb or fingers around the injured area, pressing down into injured tendons and ligaments. For example, if your ankle is sprained, circular press around the ankle joint, using the appropriate liniment. In cases of tendonitis, press only to the depth of the tendons and make small, circular movements with the thumb.

3. Finish by stroking the area to further warm and relax the muscles and stimulate circulation.

FRACTURES AND SUSPECTED FRACTURES

The main focus of any treatment of fractures with massage is to reduce swelling and inflammation while promoting free flow of qi and blood. Gentle massage above and below the site of the break is very helpful to reduce swelling and restore the free flow of circulation. If the break is severe, only light stroking movements may be tolerable. Pressure on acupressure points and ear points can be used to kill pain and stimulate the body's healing response.

Massage is only part of the treatment of fractures (see chapter 4) and should be performed only after a visit to a medical professional. If there is any doubt as to the severity of the break, do not perform massage. Do not massage open or compound fractures, and do not massage over the site of the break.

CHAPTER 15

Internal Herbal Formulas

Herbal formulas that are ingested are considered to be part of internal medicine. They are usually designed specifically for an individual so that that person's unique situation is treated appropriately. Herbs are medicinal substances and as such should be taken carefully, with attention to any unwanted side effects. *The herbal formulas in this section are presented specifically for the treatment of sports injuries, not for any other condition.* I have chosen formulas that can be used safely by a wide variety of people, but even so they should be taken only by healthy individuals who are not on medication. You should not take these formulas without consulting a licensed practitioner of traditional Chinese medicine if you

- are pregnant.

- are nursing.

- are on medication—especially anti-inflammatories and blood thinners.

- are subject to dizziness or fainting.

- are diabetic.

- are a hemophiliac.

- have lupus or other diseases of the blood.

- have cancer.

- are HIV-positive.

- have heart problems or problems of the circulatory system.

- experience excessive and prolonged bleeding during your menses.

One important thing to keep in mind about taking herbal formulas is that their actions are generally not specific to an area of the body. That is, if your knee is injured, the action of the formula is not directed specifically toward the knee. Therefore, to get the best results they should be used in conjunction with treatment of the injured area using liniments, poultices, plasters, massage, and acupressure. This helps to direct the body's energy to the injury. The exception to this is the rib fracture formula, which contains herbs that specifically direct the formula's action to the ribs.

HERBAL FORMULAS FOR ACUTE INJURY

Trauma Pills

Trauma pills (die da wan) are the internal counterpart to trauma liniment (chapter 10). Trauma pills are *the* all-purpose remedy for falls, contusions, sprains, and fractures. Most kung fu schools keep a jar of trauma pills on hand for the injuries that accompany hard training. Trauma pills clear blockages of qi, blood, and fluids that have accumulated at the site of the injury, preventing blood from congealing in the tissues of the injured area. By helping the body remove these blockages, trauma pills facilitate the return of normal circulation, allowing the injury to heal. Trauma pills strongly break stagnation. They are not for long-term use (in most cases, 2 pills a day for 2–3 days is the recommended dosage) and are not generally used for minor bruises, contusions, or muscle strains; for these injuries, trauma liniment is usually enough. Furthermore, they cannot be taken by pregnant women.

Trauma pills should be taken during the first 24–36 hours of a sprain or during the first week after a fracture or serious contusion (after this period, other formulas are more appropriate). Therefore, they are a must for your first-aid kit—you want to have them when you need them. Trauma pills can be made at home or bought at a Chinese pharmacy. Generally the homemade pills are better, as the premade, patent-medicine variety use a weaker version of the original formula.

The patent trauma pills that I recommend come in two different forms. Both forms are under the Wu Yang brand and can be purchased individually or in boxes of 12:

1. Packaged as Tieh Ta Wan, each pill comes in its own box. Inside the box is a wax ball. Break open the ball and 1 herbal pill is inside, wrapped in plastic wrap. The pill is a large ball of herbs that have been cooked in honey. Unwrap the pill, chew it up, and wash it down with warm water. Take 1 pill twice a day for 2–3 days.

2. Packaged as Circuherb Tea Extract, each wax ball contains a plastic container with a number of small black pills inside. Take all the pills inside the plastic container, with warm water. This constitutes 1 dose. Take 2 doses a day for 2–3 days.

Alternatively, you can make your own trauma pills by using the following recipe and instructions for making herbal pills with honey.

TRAUMA PILLS

10 grams	Dang gui	*Radix angelicae sinensis* (tang kuei)
10 grams	Chuan xiong	*Radix ligustici wallichii* (lovage root)
20 grams	Ru xiang	*Gummi olibanum* (frankincense)
10 grams	Mo yao	*Myrrha* (myrrh)
10 grams	Yu jin	*Tuber curcumae* (turmeric tuber)

10 grams	Tu bie chong	*Eupolyphagae seu opisthoplatiae* (wingless cockroach)*
10 grams	Zi ran tong	*Pyritium* (pyrite)
20 grams	Ma huang	*Herba ephedrae* (ephedra)

Do not take trauma pills if you are pregnant or nursing.

Do not take trauma pills if you suspect a large contusion or fracture is accompanied by internal bleeding or if there is obvious bleeding or blood loss. In these instances, use yunnan paiyao (chapter 8).

This recipe will make 50–75 trauma pills. Have the herbs ground to a fine powder by a Chinese pharmacy or herb supply company and follow the instructions on page 235 to make pills.

Dosage: Take 2 pills a day for 2–3 days.

Resinall K

An alternative to trauma pills is Resinall K, which is produced by Health Concerns, a California-based herb company. Resinall K is a modern version of an ancient injury formula. In the original formula (qi li san), the herbs were powdered and a small amount of the powder was taken with wine. In keeping with this idea, Resinall K comes as an alcohol extract. The alcohol helps the formula assimilate more quickly and aids the herbs in circulating the qi and the blood. Resinall K is not as strong as a trauma pill, but many people prefer it because of its convenient packaging. A small 1-ounce bottle will last about a week. Take ½ dropper 2 times a day for 2–3 days.

FRACTURES

Fractures heal in three distinct stages, discussed in detail in chapter 4. (If you haven't read chapter 4, go back and read it now.) During

---

* It is possible to substitute two other herbs to take the place of tu bie chong (although they do not exactly duplicate its action):

| 10 grams | Lu lu tong | *Fructus liquidambaris taiwanianae* |
| 10 grams | Chi shao | *Radix paeoniae rubra* (red peony) |

the first two weeks of a fracture (the acute phase), there is usually swelling and pain. At this time, trauma pills and Resinall K are the treatments of choice.

Rib Fracture Formula

Resinall K and trauma pills can also be used for fractured ribs; however, the rib fracture formula tends to work better because it is composed of herbs that specifically target the rib and chest area. A fractured rib can be extremely painful; sneezing, laughing, and

Making Herbal Pills with Honey

1. Have the herbs ground to a fine powder.

2. Bring honey to a boil in a pot or large frying pan. Let the honey boil for several minutes until it is liquefied.

3. Stir in the powdered herbs a little at a time until the herb-and-honey mixture has the consistency of dough.

4. Use vegetable oil to grease a large cookie sheet. Oil your hands as well to prevent the herbal mixture from sticking to them.

5. Put the herbal mixture on the cookie sheet and knead it like dough as it cools. Be careful not to burn yourself.

6. Roll out the herbal mixture into long rolls.

7. Pick off sections of the roll and form them into balls the size of large marbles.

8. Wrap each pill in waxed paper and store in a cool, dry place.

Note: Since making pills is a bit time-consuming, I recommend making a large amount that will last for a long time. Cooking the herbs with honey preserves them if they are kept out of the sunlight. For long-term storage, keep the pills in the refrigerator.

even breathing can be excruciating. Often it is uncomfortable to sleep lying down, as this puts pressure on the fracture. Broken ribs are not usually treated in Western medicine, except with painkillers, unless the rib is completely broken or impinges on the lung or another internal organ. If you know your rib is fractured and there are no complications (such as the rib puncturing the lung), taking rib fracture formula can significantly reduce the pain, ease your breathing, and help speed the healing time, especially if used in conjunction with yunnan paiyao plaster or Wu Yang pain-relieving plaster.

The rib fracture formula can also be used when intercostal muscles (the muscles between the ribs) are damaged from an impact injury. This is a common martial arts injury. The nerves in this area are very sensitive, and the pain can feel almost exactly the

Ma Huang

The herb ma huang (ephedra) has recently come under the scrutiny of the Food and Drug Administration because of deaths attributed to its presence in diet pills. Using ma huang to lose weight is an ignorant abuse of a very valuable herb. Traditionally, ma huang was never used for this purpose. It is usually prescribed for a short time only in people who are not starving themselves of nutrients and fluids. In Chinese medicine, ma huang is prescribed with other herbs for bronchial asthma because of its ability to disperse cold and dilate the bronchioles in order to stop wheezing. It is also used to treat the flu and common cold when there is coughing and wheezing. Ma huang is never used alone for these purposes. It is combined with other herbs that aid its primary action and counteract unwanted side effects.

Ma huang is sometimes included in formulas that treat sports injuries and arthritis because it opens up the tissues between the skin and the muscles and guides the other herbs of the formula into the muscles. For this reason, it is included in trauma pills. Trauma pills should be taken for 2–3 days only to help reduce the initial swelling and pain that are often associated with the acute phase of sports injuries.

same as the pain from a broken rib. This formula should be used only for rib pain resulting from an injury; it should not be used for rib pain due to internal causes such as a cough, lung abscess, lung cancer, and the like.

RIB FRACTURE FORMULA

12 grams	Dan shen	*Radix salviae miltiorrhizae* (salvia)
9 grams	Qing pi	*Pericarpium citri reticulatae viride* (immature tangerine peel)
9 grams	Chenpi	*Pericarpium citri reticulatae viride* (dried tangerine peel)
9 grams	mo yao	*Myrrha* (myrrh)
9 grams	Zhi shi	*Fructus citri seu ponciri immaturus* (bitter orange)
9 grams	Xiang fu	*Rhizoma cyperi rotundi* (nut grass rhizome)
9 grams	Chuan lain zi	*Fructus meliae toosendan* (pagoda tree fruit)
9 grams	Chai hu	*Radix bupleuri* (bupleurum)
9 grams	Lulu tong	*Fructus liquidambaris taiwanianae*
6 grams	Mu xiang	*Radix saussureae seu vladimirae* (costus root)
6 grams	Yan hu suo	*Rhizoma corydalis* (corydalis)

This formula makes 1 package of herbs. Decoct the herbs by cooking with water to make a tea. Take 1 cup of tea twice a day for 3–4 days. *Do not take*

- if the rib has punctured the lung.

- if you are pregnant or nursing.

- if you suspect there is internal bleeding.

Bone-Knitting Powder

By the second week after a fracture, the swelling and inflammation should be gone or greatly reduced if treatment was correct in the acute stage. At this point, the bone is knitting. During this phase, lasting 2–3 weeks, bone-knitting powder can be invaluable in helping the bone mend completely and without complications. Bone-kitting powder has been used for centuries by martial arts physicians and the warrior monks of Shaolin to treat injuries sustained in training and combat. This formula is particularly useful when the bone is not healing either because the damage was very extensive or because the body's resources are too depleted. The

Making Herbal Decoctions

Many herbal formulas contain dried roots and other parts of plants that are not easily digested by human beings. Extracting herbs in alcohol or powdering them makes them easier to assimilate. Another way to take herbs is to make a strong tea by cooking them with water. This is known as a "decoction." Some formulas like the rib fracture formula are more easily assimilated if prepared in this way. To make an herbal decoction:

1. Place 1 package of herbs in a stainless-steel, glass, or porcelain cooking pot. Add 4 cups of water. Cover the pot and bring to a boil.

2. When the water is boiling, reduce the flame and simmer for 35–40 minutes with the pot covered. Leave the top slightly ajar so that steam can escape.

3. Strain out the liquid and store it in a jar or bowl. Set this aside.

4. Now add three cups of liquid to the same herbs that were just cooked. Again, bring the herbs to a boil and simmer in a covered pot, with the lid slightly ajar, this time for thirty minutes.

5. Strain out the liquid and mix it with the liquid you set aside from the first cooking. You should have 2–3 cups of liquid. The herbs themselves can now be thrown away.

6. You can store the liquid in a jar in the refrigerator and warm it up to drink as a tea.

Drink 1–2 cups per day between meals.

herbs in bone-knitting powder that specifically strengthen the bones also strengthen the tendons and ligaments. For this reason, bone-knitting powder can also be used to treat recurring sprains due to overstretched ligaments.

I have given bone-knitting powder to a number of people with joints that have been injured repeatedly. The ligaments and tendons that stabilize the joint become overstretched. The joint eventually becomes too loose and clicks in and out of place constantly. This is a common injury in martial arts that emphasize joint locks. If practiced too often, joint locks gradually overstretch and tear the tissues that stabilize the joint. The wrist joint, which comprises many small bones and ligaments, is particularly susceptible to this type of injury. In these cases, bone-knitting powder can help the joint regain its stability because it contains herbs that nourish blood and strengthen the tendons and ligaments.

BONE-KNITTING POWDER

30 grams	Dang gui	*Radix angelicae sinensis* (tang kuei tails)
15 grams	Chuan xiong	*Radix ligustici wallichii* (lovage root)
15 grams	Bai shao	*Radix paeoniae alba* (white peony)
15 grams	Shu di huang	*Radix rehmanniae glutinosae conquitae* (cooked Chinese foxglove root)
15 grams	Du zhong	*Cortex eucommiae ulmoidis* (eucommia bark)
30 grams	Wu jia pi	*Cortex acanthopanacis radicis*
45 grams	Gu sui bu	*Rhizoma gusuibu* (drynaria)
15 grams	San qi	*Radix pseudoginseng* (pseudoginseng root)
15 grams	Hu gu	*Os tigris* (tiger bone)*

---

* The traditional recipe calls for tiger bone. As tigers are an endangered species, this herb is generally replaced with dog or cat bone. Many modern herbalists simply leave this ingredient out altogether and feel that its absence does not diminish the efficacy of the formula, although 30 grams of pulverized powdered chicken bone can be substituted.

30 grams	Bu gu zhi	*Fructus psoraleae corylifoliae* (scuffy pea)
30 grams	Tu si zi	*Semen cuscutae* (dodder seed)
30 grams	Dang shen	*Radix codonopsis pilosulae*
15 grams	Mu gua	*Fructus chaenomelis lagenariae* (quince fruit)
30 grams	Liu ji nu	*Herba artemisiae anomalae*
45 grams	Tu bie chong	*Eupolyphagae seu opisthopatiae* (wingless cockroach)*
15 grams	Huang qi	*Radix astragali seu hedysari* (astragalus root)
15 grams	Dang shen	*Radix codonopsis pilosulae*
30 grams	Xu duan	*Radix dipsaci* (Japanese teasel root)

Have the herbs ground to a fine powder. Take ¼ teaspoon 2 times a day, or make honey pills (see "Making Herbal Pills with Honey") and take 1 pill twice a day. Take bone-knitting powder for 2–3 weeks during the knitting stage and complete healing stage of fracture healing (see chapter 4).

BONE SPURS

Bone spurs are most likely to manifest in people over forty. They are often associated with chronic inflammation of a joint, tendonitis, and arthritis. Chronic inflammation can cause calcium to be deposited at the margins of a joint or where an inflamed tendon attaches to the bone. Over time, an outgrowth of bone, called an "osteophyte," may develop. Osteophytes occur most commonly on the heel but can also form in the shoulder, neck, spine, and hip. Because these bony projections are often sharp or pointed in shape, they are known as "bone spurs." Bone spurs can be difficult to treat. They can irritate surrounding tissues, leading to pain and weakness and eventually disuse and atrophy.

---

* There is no real substitute for this herb in this formula; however, 30 grams of zi ran tong (*Pyritium;* pyrite) can be used instead.

Clinical studies in China have shown that traditional Chinese medicine can eliminate symptoms of pain and weakness and inhibit the growth of new spurs. Acupuncture in conjunction with herbal soaks and plasters can be effective in treating bone spurs, but the effectiveness is increased when these therapies are supported by ingestion of herbs internally. One internal herbal formula that is very effective for bone spurs is osteophyte powder. My colleagues and I have recommended osteophyte powder to many people with bone spurs in the neck, spine, shoulder, and heel. In some cases, pain and weakness diminished after as little as 2 weeks. On the average, the powder needs to be taken for 2–3 months to see results.

Chinese Herbs vs. Western Herbs

When using the herbal formulas in this book, order the herbs from a reputable Chinese herb store—a number of these are listed in appendix 2. Do not try to replace the ingredients with Western herbs that sound similar or are from the same family of plants. Chinese herbs have specific properties that are a reflection of

- where the plant was grown.

- what soil and climate it was grown in.

- when the herb was harvested.

- how the herb was prepared—dried, steamed, precooked, and so on.

- how it synergistically interacts with the other herbs in the formula.

Western herbs are also very effective, but they are prescribed according to different theories and are often prepared and harvested differently. Only a qualified expert in both systems is capable of making the appropriate substitutions.

OSTEOPHYTE POWDER

30 grams	Shu di huang	*Radix rehmanniae glutinosae conquitae* (cooked Chinese foxglove root)
30 grams	Lu xian cao	*Herba pyrolae rotundifloiae*
30 grams	Gu sui bu	*Rhizoma guisuibu* (drynaria)
30 grams	Rou cong rong	*Herba cistanches* (cistanchis)
30 grams	Ji xue teng	*Radix et caulis jixueteng* (millettia root and vine)
30 grams	Yin yang huo	*Herba epimedii* (epimedium)
30 grams	Lai fu zi	*Semen raphani sativi* (radish seed)

Do not take if pregnant or nursing.

Take ¼ teaspoon of powder 2 times a day with warm water, or make honey pills (see "Making Herbal Pills with Honey") and take 1 pill 2 times a day.

Interactions Between Chinese Herbs and Western Drugs

Herbal formulas for sports injuries are usually taken for a short period of time, so negative side effects or unwanted interactions with Western drugs are not usually an issue. However, there are several circumstances in which these formulas *cannot* be taken with certain Western drugs or should be taken with care under the supervision of a licensed practitioner of traditional Chinese medicine who is communicating with your doctor. Whenever you ingest Chinese herbs, if unusual symptoms develop, stop taking the herbs and symptoms will usually disappear fairly quickly.

ANTI-INFLAMMATORIES AND ANTIBIOTICS

Anti-inflammatories often irritate the stomach, and antibiotics upset some people's intestinal function. The majority of the herbs used in

Chinese medicine are derived from plants. Many Chinese herbs are roots, which can be difficult for the digestive tract of human beings to break down and assimilate. Cooking herbs with water or alcohol extracts or powdering the herbs makes them easier to assimilate, but they can tax the digestive system if combined with anti-inflammatories or antibiotics.

BLOOD THINNERS

Drugs that thin the blood often interact with the herbal formulas used in Chinese sports medicine. Herbal formulas that treat trauma contain herbs that are said to "move the blood," aiding the blocked or retarded circulation that occurs in the injured area. These formulas also break up accumulations of qi and blood to prevent blood from congealing in the local tissues. Blood thinners prevent clots from forming in the blood vessels, so their action is somewhat similar to that of blood-moving herbs. Blood thinners are very strong drugs whose dosage must be monitored carefully. In combination with blood-moving herbs, their effect on the body is too strong, making a person feel dizzy or faint. There is also potential for such a combination to interfere with normal clotting of the blood.

SEIZURE MEDICATION

Seizure medications affect brain function and can produce many strange side effects. Their interactions with Chinese herbs are not well understood, so to be on the safe side it is best not to take them at the same time without supervision.

HEART MEDICATIONS

Both heart medications and herbal formulas used to treat trauma affect the circulation of the blood. Heart medications regulate heart function, thereby creating global effects on the body's circulation. Although Chinese herbs work differently, in combination with heart medications, there can be unwanted side effects.

CHAPTER 16

Moxibustion

In earlier chapters, I have advocated therapies that make use of heat—warming herbs, hot herbal soaks, and wet heat in the form of hydrocollator packs. These therapies are invaluable for restoring normal circulation to injured areas and encouraging the reabsorption of pockets of stagnant blood and fluids that often remain when the injury is no longer acute. Moxibustion is a unique form of heat therapy used for centuries by acupuncturists. In the past, moxibustion was often used alone as an independent therapy. Today it is considered to be part of the practice of acupuncture. The term *zhen jiu,* which is often translated into English as "acupuncture," actually refers to both therapies. *Zhen* means to puncture the body with a needle, and *jiu* refers to using fire to heat acupoints.

Moxibustion involves burning the dried leaves of the mugwort plant (ai ye; *Folium artemisiae*) to produce a penetrating heat. This heat can be directed into acupuncture points, muscles, or joints. Traditionally, this was done in three ways:

1. The dried leaves are formed into small cones, which are burned directly on the skin over acupuncture points. This method is very powerful, because it creates an intense heat that penetrates the point, bringing with it the volatile oils contained in the leaf. Often, small scars result from this

procedure, which is why this method is not used extensively today.

2. The dried leaves are formed into balls that are placed on the handles of acupuncture needles. The heat is conducted through the needle and into the point. This method is frequently employed by acupuncturists.

3. The skin is heated indirectly with a moxa pole. Moxa poles are large cigars of rolled mugwort that are lit and held near the skin. This allows the radiant heat to penetrate joints, muscles, and acupoints. This is the method most often used by martial arts practitioners to treat sports injuries and the method that will be described here.

Moxa poles have a wide range of applications in the treatment of sports injuries. Heating injured areas with the moxa pole allows the oils in the smoke to contact the skin. These oils actually enhance the effect of the radiant heat produced by the burning pole. The oils penetrate the meridians and local tissues, creating additional warming and blood-activating effects independent of the radiant heat.

Studies in China have shown that moxibustion using a moxa stick increases blood circulation and disperses accumulations of stagnant blood more effectively than other forms of radiant heat. These effects are strongest if the injured area is fumigated with the smoke, thereby allowing the oils in the smoke to penetrate.

Moxibustion is generally used in the postacute phase of sports injuries, after the initial inflammation is gone and the swelling is significantly reduced. In fractures, moxibustion is used during the complete healing stage of treatment (see chapter 4).

Moxibustion can be used

- to help reduce residual swelling, pain, and stiffness.

- to disperse remaining accumulations of stagnant blood and fluids.

- to warm injured areas that are cold to the touch, indicating inadequate circulation, or when chronic injuries ache in cold, damp weather.

I treated a patient with chronic knee pain. Acupuncture, massage, and other therapies had helped but not resolved the problem. I noticed his knee was very cold to the touch. I had my assistant heat the knee with moxibustion, but even after several minutes he did not really feel the warmth and the knee itself would not hold any heat for more than a few seconds. I lit a second stick and began to heat the KID 1 (chapter 7) acupoint on the bottom of the foot. I heated the point for thirty seconds, then pressed the heat into the point for several seconds. The two of us heated his leg for thirty minutes before he began to feel the warmth. By forty minutes he could feel the warmth throughout his whole lower leg. His knee immediately felt much better. We gave him several moxa sticks to continue the treatment at home, and that completed his recovery.

Moxibustion should not be used (or used with great caution)

- over skin ulcerations or open lesions.

- in any situation in which skin sensitivity is diminished.

- over the lower back or abdomen of a pregnant woman.

- on points such as LI 4, ST 36, or the tip of the little toe if you are pregnant.

- when an injured area is hot, red, and painful.

USING MOXA POLES

After the moxa pole is lit, blow on it softly as you let it burn, until the tip forms into a round shape. As you use the pole, you will need to tap the ash into an ashtray periodically. An air purifier or ionizer can help reduce the smell and smoke if you are indoors.

Heating the Injured Area

When using a moxa pole, heat the injured area slowly by moving the tip of the lit pole in small circles over the injured area. Keep the pole at a distance that is warm and comfortable. The idea is to create a warm, spreading heat that builds over 5–10 minutes. Continue until the area is pink or slightly red. Holding the pole too close to the skin too soon will heat the skin quickly, creating an uncomfortable burning sensation and reducing the therapeutic effect. Moxibustion can be used in conjunction with warming liniments such as U-I oil and tendon lotion (chapter 11). This combination helps the liniments to penetrate the tissues, increasing their effect. Do not follow moxibustion immediately with warming medicated plasters. Let the skin cool first to prevent causing a burn.

Heating Acupoints

Acupoints like ST 36 and LI 10 (chapter 13) can be stimulated with a moxa pole. This is particularly useful when the injured area is cold or weak. For example, if you have chronic knee pain, and the knee is stiff, weak, and susceptible to the cold, use the moxa pole to stimulate ST 36. To stimulate an acupoint like ST 36 with a moxa pole, move the pole close to the point and then quickly pull it away, like a sparrow pecking at crumbs. Repeat this motion, slowly heating the point until it becomes slightly red over a 5–10-minute period. This creates a sensation of the heat being pushed or pressed into the point.

Extinguishing the Moxa Pole

It can be difficult to extinguish a moxa pole. It should be smothered by placing the tip in sand or salt. Moxa extinguishers can be purchased from many herb stores and acupuncture supply companies, although wrapping the tip in tinfoil works just as well. Do not wet the moxa pole to extinguish it, as moisture can ruin the pole. If possible, moxa poles should be stored in a dry, cool place away from moisture and humidity.

COMMON USES OF MOXIBUSTION

Jammed Finger

Moxibustion can be very useful in treating jammed fingers after the initial swelling is gone or reduced. The joints of the fingers are encased in a tight joint capsule. Once stagnant blood and fluids have accumulated in the joint, it can be difficult to restore normal circulation inside the joint. Bleeding, herbal soaks, and liniments can remove most of these stagnant fluids, but often some accumulation remains. Moxibustion helps to alleviate the residual stiffness that often remains in the joint, preventing complete range of motion. For best results, hold the finger over the stick so that the smoke fumigates the joint.

When I taught Filipino stick fighting (*eskrima*), I treated many finger joints that were chronically injured from strikes to the hand. In almost every case, moxibustion removed the stiffness that prevented complete bending of the joints.

Sprained Ankle

The swelling associated with an ankle sprain can linger for months afterward. This residual swelling, even if slight, indicates that normal circulation has not been completely restored to the injured tissues. Heat acupoints ST 36 and GB 39 (chapter 13) with a moxa pole and then slowly heat the ankle until it is pink or the swelling is visibly reduced.

Chronic Knee Pain

Use moxibustion if you have chronic knee pain, particularly when the pain increases with cold, damp weather. Heat ST 36 with the moxa pole and then slowly heat the knee itself.

Back Pain

Moxibustion is very effective for chronic back pain, especially when the back is stiff and sore in cold or damp weather. First heat the painful area and then use the moxa pole to heat the dimples in the lower back. These are special acupoints where the heat can penetrate deeply into the back muscles. Applying U-I oil (Chapter 10) after warming the back with a moxa pole can increase the effectiveness of the treatment, because one of the ingredients in U-I oil is mugwort oil, extracted from the same leaves that are in the moxa pole. *Caution:* Do not use moxibustion on the back of the knee or on the BL 40 acupoint, as this can increase tension in the tendons behind the knee.

Neck Pain

One of my friends got a stiff neck several times last year. The first time, he slept with air-conditioning blowing on him. Several months later, he put an ice-cold towel around his neck because he was hot and sweaty. Then in the winter he was out in the cold after he had eaten a lot of spicy food that made him sweat. In each case, his neck pain was due to the cold penetrating the neck through the open pores of the skin. In Chinese medicine, the back of the neck is considered to be particularly sensitive to attack by the elements. If you are sweating and then exposed to a cold wind, you are even more susceptible to the penetration of cold. Fortunately, heat in the form of moxibustion can activate the circulation and drive out the cold. This is how we treated my friend's neck. First heat the back of the neck. Then heat the point that is just below the seventh cervical vertebra (the big bump at the base of the neck). Finally, heat two points that are about a thumb's width off the midline of the neck. They are small hollows that are easy to see near the base of the neck. Applications of wet heat in the form of a hydrocollator pack or hot towels can also be helpful.

Treatments for Common Sports Injuries and Miscellaneous Injuries

INTRODUCTION TO PART IV

This section is a quick reference guide to common sports injuries. As it is not possible to cover every injury that could possibly occur, the most common injuries or those that are representative of how to treat a group of similar conditions will be listed. Many of the specific treatments and remedies mentioned in this section are discussed in detail earlier in the book, in parts 1 and 3. Whenever possible, they are presented in **bold print**. The reader is advised to then go to that section of the book for a more complete discussion of how and when to use the remedy. Many of the rehabilitative exercises mentioned are covered in part 2. Whenever an exercise is recommended that is not in part 2, it will be explained in this section.

The components of herbal formulas are listed in part 3. Appendix 2 lists sources from which you can purchase herbal remedies by mail order. For those who may need to use these remedies frequently, or want to incorporate them as part of their training routine, appendix 1 presents a basic Chinese sports medicine first-aid kit that is inexpensive to put together and can effectively treat most of the conditions listed in this section.

Each listing in this section contains the following headings:

First aid: This section discusses what to do first. For a fresh acute injury, it is literally a first-aid treatment aimed at reducing swelling, pain, and inflammation. For a more chronic injury such as a bone spur, this section will tell you which remedies to try first.

Follow-up treatment: This section covers treatments to use after the first-aid stage, when swelling, pain, and inflammation are reduced, until resuming the sport or activity.

Exercises: These include both specific exercises to rehabilitate the injury so that activity can be resumed and sets of exercises that strengthen the body or increase its flexibility to prevent reinjury. (Sets of exercises are found in chapters 5 and 6.)

Acupoints and massage: Self-massage techniques can be used alone or with liniments, as well as with ear acupoints that can be stimulated by taping a small seed over the point. (See chapters 13 and 14.)

Diet: This section covers dietary dos and don'ts specific to the injury. Detailed discussion of these can be found in chapter 7.

Important:

1. Chinese sports medicine works best when multiple therapies are used to address different aspects of an injury. Therefore, internal and external use of herbs in combination with physical techniques like massage, moxibustion, or cupping and rehabilitative exercise and diet produce the best results. Do go back and read the earlier chapters that detail how to use these therapies.

2. When using plasters, poultices, and liniments, always clean the area thoroughly and allow time in between for the skin to breathe when switching from one plaster or liniment to another. Otherwise there can be interactions among the herbal constituents. If a rash develops, discontinue or decrease use.

3. If you are in doubt about the nature of your injury or its severity, consult a physician.

Treatments

ACHILLES' TENDONITIS

This is inflammation of the Achilles' tendon. Achilles' tendonitis is usually caused by overuse or improper use of the leg or ankle, although it can also be caused by a blow to the ankle, the calf muscle, or the tendon itself. Tendonitis is often the result of repeated injury. Inflammation of the tendon causes it to swell in its sheath, creating further irritation. The tendon often looks or feels thicker than the other side (this is due to the swelling) and may be red and hot to the touch (the inflammation). The ankle may feel stiff, and range of motion may be limited. A crackling or creaking sound may occur when the foot and ankle are flexed and extended.

First Aid

1. If the tendon is red and warm to the touch, mix **san huang san** (chapter 11) with Vaseline or green tea and apply to the local area. Leave on for 24–48 hours. If necessary, cover the calf muscle with san huang san. Alternatively, apply the **Wu Yang pain-relieving plaster** (chapter 11).

2. Massage the back of the knee, the calf, and the Achilles' tendon with **trauma liniment** (chapter 10).

3. Press the **GB 39** acupoint and the **heel pain point** on the hand to relieve pain (chapter 13).

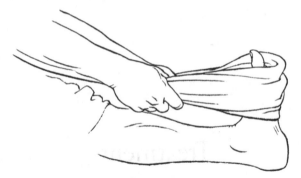

Figure 126.

Follow-up Treatment

1. If inflammation and heat are gone, massage the calf and the Achilles' tendon with **tendon lotion** (chapter 10).

2. Use the **tendon-relaxing soak** (chapter 12) twice a day for 1–2 weeks.

3. Before and after stretching or exercising, apply **tendon lotion, Chinese Massage Oil,** or **U-I oil** (chapter 10).

Exercises

1. Do the **Daily Dozen** (chapter 5) to improve flexibility and prevent reinjury, especially **Knee Rotation** and **Phoenix Stretch.**

2. Gently stretch the Achilles' tendon by pulling on the toes or doing the towel stretch. Hook a towel over the ball of your foot and gently pull the foot toward you to stretch the Achilles' tendon. (Figure 126.) Repeat several times on each leg. Do the towel stretch every day until the injury is fully healed.

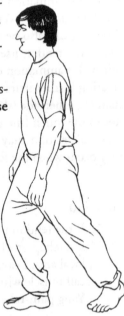

Figure 127.

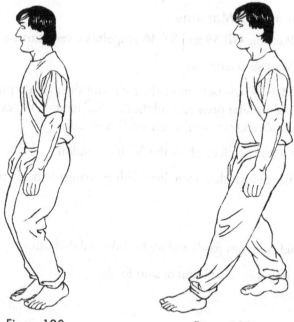

Figure 128.   Figure 129.

3. As the inflammation lessens, progress to the slow walk exercise, taking a step as slowly as possible. Try to lift the rear
foot all at once from inside the hip joint, so that someone
standing behind you cannot see the heel rise. (Figure 127.)
Then very slowly bring that foot forward, with the sole of
the foot slightly off the floor. (Figure 128.) Be careful not to
let the supporting leg shake or to lean to one side. Keep the
hips and head centered. Try to take 1 minute to take a single step. Set the foot down lightly, placing the entire sole of
the foot on the floor. (Figure 129.) Repeat on the other
side. Take 3–5 steps on each leg. Do this exercise twice a
day until the injury is fully healed and you have resumed
normal activities. This exercise is very important in the
rehabilitation of many leg injuries.

Acupoints and Massage

1. Press the **GB 39** and **ST 36** acupoints several times a day.

2. Massage treatment:

   • Massage the bottom of the foot, and then gently **press** and **circular press** around the Achilles' tendon. Put extra emphasis on areas that are swollen or hard.

   • Gently pinch or pluck the Achilles' tendon.

3. **Ear points:** shen men, liver, kidney, sympathetic, heel.

Diet

   • Avoid cold, raw foods and iced drinks and shellfish.

   • Eat only a small amount of sour foods.

ANKLE SPRAIN

One of the most common sports injuries, ankle sprains typically occur when the foot is rolled inward, stretching and tearing the ligaments on the outside of the ankle. In a mild sprain, the ligaments that hold the bones of the ankle together are stretched and sometimes slightly torn. In a severe sprain, one or more ligaments are completely torn. This ligament damage can create instability in the joint, making it susceptible to further injury if the sprain is treated improperly or not fully healed. Severe sprains with ligaments that are completely torn may require surgical repair.

First Aid

1. Bleed and cup the area to reduce swelling and blood stagnation.

2. Massage **trauma liniment** (chapter 10) into the ankle and foot. Massage lightly over the swollen, black-and-blue area and more deeply above and below the sprain.

3. Press **GB 34** and **GB 39**. Press **ST 31** and **ST 36** (chapter 13).

4. Mix **san huang san** (chapter 11) with green tea or Vaseline and apply to the ankle while it is swollen, to reduce swelling and inflammation.

5. Take a **trauma pill** twice a day for 2–3 days. Alternatively, take **Resinall K** twice a day for 2–3 days (chapter 15).

6. Elevate the foot to further reduce the swelling.

7. Perform simple range-of-motion exercises that do not aggravate the injury. If the sprain is severe, these may have to wait until there is less pain.

Follow-up Treatment

1. Massage with **trauma liniment** (chapter 10) directly over the site of the injury. Push with the palm and the thumb from the sprained area up the leg and from below the sprained area to the tips of the toes. This helps stagnant fluids and blood to be reabsorbed.

2. Soak the ankle in the **tendon-relaxing soak** (chapter 12) to relax spasms in the tendons and muscles that are inhibiting range of motion.

3. If pain and stiffness are worse with the cold, massage **tendon lotion** or **U-I oil** (chapter 10) into the injured area.

4. Use a moxa stick to warm the area and help reduce any residual swelling (chapter 16). Moxa **ST 36** and **GB 39**.

Exercises

1. Pick up a towel with your toes and turn the ankle inward and outward. (Figure 130.)

2. While seated, lift the foot slightly off the floor and draw letters in the air with your foot. Allow the toes to point and flex as you draw the letters.

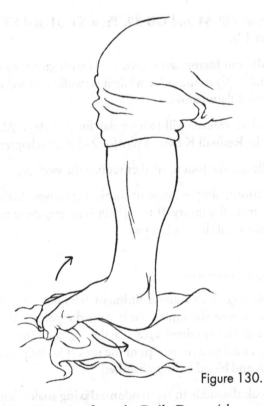

Figure 130.

3. Do **Knee Rotation** from the **Daily Dozen** (chapter 5).

4. As the ankle gets stronger, do the **slow walk exercise** (see "Achilles' Tendonitis").

Acupoints and Massage

1. Press **ST 31, ST 36, GB 34,** and **GB 39.**

2. Massage treatment:

- **Press** and **circular press** with the thumb around the ankle bones.

- **Grasp** the calf muscle.

- **Press** and pinch the Achilles' tendon.

3. **Ear points:** ankle, liver, shen men, sympathetic.

Diet

- Avoid shellfish.
- Cut down on cold, raw foods.
- Avoid iced drinks.
- Avoid roasted or fried foods.

ARTHRITIS

Arthritis means that there is inflammation in a joint, resulting in pain and swelling. When most people talk about arthritis, what they are referring to is osteoarthritis, which is a degenerative process that usually begins in the cartilage that lines the surfaces between the bone; rheumatoid arthritis, on the other hand, is a systemic disorder associated with autoimmune dysfunction. Cartilage is thick and fibrous as well as rubbery. It allows the bones that constitute the joint to move smoothly without rubbing against one another and in joints like the knee and hip cartilage it cushions bones against compressive forces.

Although osteoarthritis often manifests in middle age, it is not just a result of the aging process. Osteoarthritis is usually due to chronically overloading or overstressing a joint or a misalignment of the body, which forces undue stress on one of the joints. It can also be the result of a previous injury involving damaged cartilage or damage to joint structures. In either case, the cartilage becomes worn, causing the bones to rub together. This creates inflammation. Chronic inflammation of the joint causes normal tissue to be replaced with thick fibrous tissue. It can also inhibit normal circulation to the bones and the underlying cartilage. The undernourished tissue wears away and the margins of the joint can deform, causing projections of bone or spurs. Ultimately, the joint is chronically painful and more restricted in its range of motion. Osteoarthritis can occur in the spine, knee, elbow, shoulder, fingers, or any joint that is chronically injured or inflamed.

First Aid

Because osteoarthritis develops over time, there is no acute phase.

Follow-up Treatment

1. Apply the **sinew-bone poultice** (chapter 11) by mixing the powdered herbs with whiskey or rice wine.

2. Apply **701 plasters, gou pi Plaster,** or **hua tuo anticontusion rheumatism plaster** (chapter 11).

3. Massage **tendon lotion** or **U-I oil** (chapter 10) into the joint. This can be followed by soaking a cloth or gauze in the liniment and wrapping it around the joint like a poultice.

4. Use the **warming soak** (chapter 12), particularly if the joint is more painful in cold, damp weather.

5. Heat the area with a moxa stick for 5–10 minutes a day until it is pink and warm (chapter 16).

Exercises

1. Exercises that maintain range of motion and strengthen muscles around the joint(s) without overstressing them can help stop degeneration of the joint. The **Daily Dozen** (chapter 5) and the **Eight Brocade Plus** (chapter 6) help the body to maintain flexibility and improve strength without irritating or inflaming joints.

2. The **health preservation exercises** (chapter 7) are invaluable for promoting circulation and the health of the internal organs.

Acupoints and Massage

1. Frequently massage the injured joint(s):

   • **Grasp** the large muscle groups above and below the joint.

- **Press** and **circular press** around the joint.

- Pay particular attention to any crevices between the bones, acupoints nearby the joint, or more distant acupoints that affect the injured area of the body (see chapter 13).

2. Ear points: shen men, sympathetic, spleen, kidney, point related to injured area.

Diet

- Reduce or avoid intake of cold, raw foods and iced drinks.

- Avoid deep-fried and fatty foods.

- Eat foods that tonify the qi and blood.

BACK SPRAIN/STRAIN—LOWER

Lower back sprains are caused by sudden forceful overstretching of the ligaments of the sacroiliac joint or the ligaments around the spine. Lower back strains occur when muscles and tendons are overstretched or torn, causing an inflammatory response. Sprains and strains in the back can become chronic when the deep muscles spasm and shorten to protect the back. Often, the abdominal muscles and the psoas muscle, a deep hip flexor that helps to stabilize the lumbar vertebrae, also go into spasm as part of the body's protective response.

First Aid

1. Do slow, abdominal breathing. Breathe into the back. The diaphragm has attachments that connect to the lumbar spine. Abdominal breathing can help keep the diaphragm from contracting, which will further tighten the tissues of the back (see chapter 5).

2. Take a **trauma pill** twice a day for 2–3 days. Alternatively, take **Resinall K** twice a day for 2–3 days (chapter 15).

3. Cup the injured area (chapter 9).

4. Apply **trauma liniment** (chapter 10) to the sore, strained area.

5. Apply **Wu Yang pain-relieving plaster** or **yunnan paiyao plaster** (chapter 11).

6. Press and massage **BL 60** and **BL 40** to relieve pain (chapter 13).

7. Rest the back, but avoid immobilizing it by lying down all day. Periodically do gentle stretching and range-of-motion exercises. To reduce pain while moving the back, press **yao tong xue** (lumbar pain point) or stimulate ear acupoints (chapter 13).

Follow-up Treatment

1. Once the inflammation is gone, soak hot towels in the **tendon-relaxing soak** (chapter 12) and apply to the lower back. Or apply more warming plasters such as **701 plasters** or **gou pi plaster** (chapter 11).

2. Continue to press and rub **BL 40** and **BL 60** or the **yao tong xue** points on the hand (chapter 13) whenever you remember throughout the day.

3. Soak in a whirlpool or hot tub after the initial inflammation is gone to relieve muscle tension and soreness.

4. If the back injury is old or chronic, get a family member or friend to heat the back with a moxa pole, followed by soaking a cloth or paper towel in **U-I oil** (chapter 10) and applying it to the back for 10 or 15 minutes. Or put hot, wet towels or a hydrocollator pack over the soaked toweling to allow the oil to penetrate the skin.

5. Rub **tendon lotion** (chapter 10) into the back several times a day.

6. Do **health preservation exercises** (chapter 7), particularly 14, 15, and 16.

Exercises

1. Do the **Daily Dozen** (chapter 5), especially **Phoenix Stretch, Hula Hips and Hip Rotation**, and **Swing the Leg to Open the Hip.**

2. Do the **Eight Brocade Plus** (chapter 6), especially **Squatting to Strengthen the Back and Legs** and **Shake the Head and Wag the Tail.**

3. Stretch the psoas muscles by stepping into a lunge position and stretching the hands up overhead. (Figure 131.) You should feel a stretch in the deep muscles in the front of the abdomen. This exercise should be done only after the acute phase of the injury has passed.

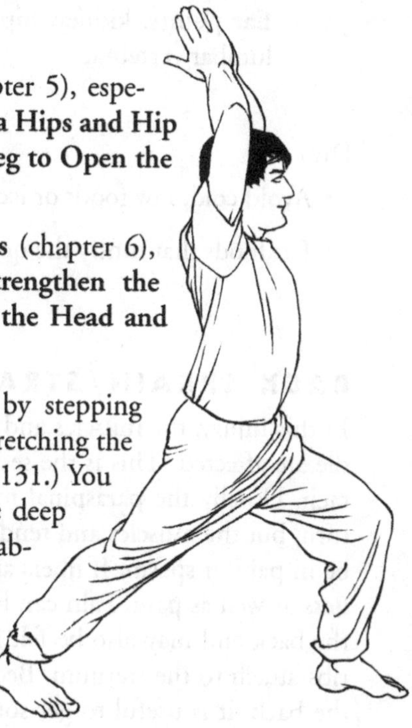

Figure 131.

4. If the sacroiliac area was strained, practice walking backward slowly, keeping the body erect. With your weight on the right foot, reach back with the left leg until the ball of the left foot touches the floor. Slowly shift the weight to the left foot. Repeat on the other side. Repeat 10–20 times per session. This strengthens the sacroiliac joint and helps to heal tears in muscles in that area.

Acupoints and Massage

1. Press the **BL 40** and **BL 60** acupoints several times a day.

2. Massage treatment:

   • **Press** and **circular press** the injured area.

   • **Palm push** down either side of the spine.

   • **Thumb push** along the sides of the sacrum.

3. **Ear points:** kidney, hip, buttock, shen men, sympathetic, lumbar vertebrae.

Diet

- Avoid cold, raw foods or iced drinks.

- Eat foods that tonify the qi and blood.

BACK SPRAIN/STRAIN—UPPER

In this injury, the muscles and tendons of the upper back or middle are affected. This is the section of the spine where the ribs attach. Usually the paraspinal muscles and tendons are strained or torn, but the muscles and tendons that attach to the ribs may also be in pain or spasm. If fibers are torn, there may be muscle weakness as well as pain. Pain can be along one or more ribs as well as the back and may also be felt in the front of the body, where the ribs attach to the sternum. Because it is hard to reach this area of the back, it is useful to get someone to help you with liniments, massage techniques, or plasters.

First Aid

1. Do slow, natural abdominal breathing to keep the diaphragm from becoming tight or going into spasm.

2. Take a **trauma pill** twice a day for 2–3 days. Alternatively, take **Resinall K** twice a day for 2–3 days (chapter 15).

3. Cup the injured area (chapter 9).

4. Apply **trauma liniment** (chapter 10) to the sore, strained area.

5. Apply **Wu Yang pain-relieving plaster** or **yunnan paiyao plaster** (chapter 11).

6. Press and massage the **BL 60** and **BL 40** acupoints to relieve pain (chapter 13).

Follow-up Treatment

1. Once the inflammation is gone, soak hot towels in the **tendon-relaxing soak** (chapter 12) and apply to the lower back, or apply more warming plasters such as **701 plasters** or **gou pi plaster** (chapter 11).

2. Continue to press and rub **BL 40** and **BL 60** whenever you remember throughout the day (chapter 13).

3. Soak in a whirlpool or hot tub after the initial inflammation is gone to relieve muscle tension and soreness.

4. If the back injury is old or chronic, get a family member or friend to heat the back with a moxa pole (chapter 16), followed by soaking a cloth or paper towel in **U-I oil** (chapter 10) and applying it to the back for 10 or 15 minutes. Or put hot, wet towels or a hydrocollator pack over the soaked toweling to allow the oil to penetrate the skin.

5. Rub **tendon lotion** (chapter 10) into the back several times a day.

Exercises

1. With the knees bent and shoulder width apart, slowly bend forward, rolling the spine downward as you exhale. When the arms are hanging all the way down (they may drag on the floor), hold and breathe for several breaths. With each exhale feel the weight of the arms pulling the ribs apart and, like an accordion, relaxing tight, strained tissues. Slowly rise as you inhale, rolling the spine upward until you are erect. Do this exercise several times a day.

2. Cross your arms so that each palm cups an elbow. With the knee slightly bent, bend the body at the waist until the arms are hanging down. Let gravity pull the ribs and upper back open and then make a circle with the arms, first going upward toward the head as you inhale and then reaching out and downward as you exhale. As the arms move downward, feel the ribs and vertebrae in the upper back gently stretch

and separate. Repeat several times in one direction and then reverse directions. (Figures 132–134.)

3. Do the **Daily Dozen** (chapter 5), especially **Arm Rotation, Elbow Rotation,** and **Sinew Stretching.**

4. Do the **Eight Brocade Plus** (chapter 6), especially **Drawing the Bow to Shoot the Eagle, Holding Up a Single Hand, Looking Backward and Twisting Like a Dragon,** and **Clenching the Fists and Glaring Increases Strength.**

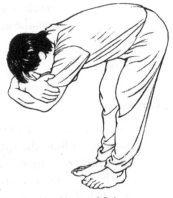

Figure 132.

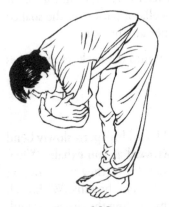

Figure 133.

Figure 134.

5. If there is chronic tightness in the upper back so that the normal curvature of the back is exaggerated and hunched over, firmly roll up a bath towel so that it is 4–6 inches thick. Lie on the towel so that its length runs across the hunched section of your back. Lie on the towel for 10–15 minutes, feeling the body progressively relax as you stretch your upper back on the towel. (Figure 135.)

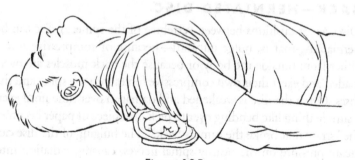

Figure 135.

Do not fall asleep on the towel, as this will overstretch the area—10–15 minutes a day is enough. When you are done, get up slowly. Avoid making any sudden movements or lifting anything heavy for several minutes.

Acupoints and Massage

1. Bend over so that the arms can reach up the back. Use the backs of the hands to rub up and down on either side of the spine.

2. It is hard to massage your upper back. If you can get a family member or friend to massage your back, have him or her **palm push** down the back for several minutes on the muscles on either side of the spine.

3. **Ear points:** shen men, sympathetic, thoracic vertebrae, liver, spleen.

Diet

- Avoid cold, raw foods or iced drinks.
- Eat foods that tonify the qi and blood.

BACK—HERNIATED DISC

Discs act as cushions between vertebrae of the spine. A disc can be herniated—that is, bulge outward—because of compressive forces either from outside the body or because the back muscles are overloaded and exert their own compressive forces into the spine and the discs. Often the disc is weakened and damaged over time until even a simple thing like bending over to pick up a piece of paper becomes the "straw that broke the camel's back." The bulging of the disc can create pressure on the nearby spinal nerves, causing radiation into the buttocks or down the back of the leg (sciatic pain). Herniated discs are most common in the lumbar spine between L4 and L5 and are common in the neck, especially in cases of whiplash. In chronic, long-standing disc problems, the disc space narrows as the disc is gradually compressed by the bone. The two vertebrae no longer work independently, thereby limiting range of motion. The vertebrae on either side of the disc can develop bone spurs because of the constant irritation, and the joint becomes arthritic.

First Aid

1. Do slow, abdominal breathing. Breathe into the back. The diaphragm has attachments that connect to the lumbar spine. Abdominal breathing can help keep the diaphragm from contracting, which will further tighten the tissues of the back (see chapter 5).

2. Take a **trauma pill** twice a day for 2–3 days. Alternatively, take **Resinall K** twice a day for 2–3 days (chapter 15).

3. Cup the injured area. If there is swelling, bleed in the swollen area alongside the spine and then cup to draw out the stagnant blood (chapter 9).

4. Apply **san huang san** (chapter 11) mixed with green tea to the area. Cover with gauze pads and wrap around the body with rolled gauze.

5. Apply **trauma liniment** (chapter 10) to the sore, strained area.

6. Apply **Wu Yang pain-relieving plaster** or **yunnan paiyao plaster** (chapter 11).

7. Press and massage the **BL 60** and **BL 40** acupoints to relieve pain (chapter 13).

8. Rest the back, but avoid immobilizing it by lying down all day. Periodically do gentle stretching and range-of-motion exercises. To reduce pain while moving the back, press **yao tong xue** (lumbar pain point) or stimulate ear acupoints (chapter 13).

Follow-up Treatment

1. Once the inflammation is gone, soak hot towels in the **tendon-relaxing soak** (chapter 12) and apply to the lower back, or apply more warming plasters such as **701 plasters** or **gou pi plaster** (chapter 11).

2. Continue to press and rub **BL 40** and **BL 60** or the **yao tong xue** points on the hand whenever you remember throughout the day (chapter 13).

3. Soak in a whirlpool or hot tub after the initial inflammation is gone to relieve muscle tension and soreness.

4. If the disc injury is old or chronic, get a family member to heat the back with a moxa pole, followed by soaking a cloth or paper towel in **U-I oil** (chapter 10) and applying it to the back for 10 or 15 minutes. Or put hot, wet towels or a hydrocollator pack over the soaked toweling to allow the oil to penetrate the skin.

5. Rub **tendon lotion** (chapter 10) into the back several times a day.

6. Do **health preservation exercises** (chapter 7), particularly 14, 15, and 16.

Exercises

1. Initially perform **Phoenix Stretch** and **Hula Hips and Hip Rotation** from the **Daily Dozen** (chapter 5).

2. Later, add **Squatting to Strengthen the Back and Legs,** from the **Eight Brocade Plus** (chapter 6). This helps to open up the lumbar area and create space between the discs.

3. Stretch the psoas muscles by stepping into a lunge position and stretching the hands up overhead. You should feel a stretch in the deep muscles in the front of the abdomen (see "Back Sprain/Strain—Lower"). This exercise should be done only after the acute phase of the injury has passed.

4. Lie on your back with the feet flat on the floor and the knees bent, and pull the knee to the chest as you keep your lumbar spine on the floor.

5. Eventually progress to doing the **Daily Dozen** (chapter 5) and the **Eight Brocade Plus** (chapter 6) to prevent reinjury.

Acupoints and Massage

1. Massage treatment:

• **Press** and **circular press** the injured area.

• **Palm push** down either side of the spine.

• **Thumb push** downward along the sides of the vertebrae that are involved.

2. **Ear points:** lumbar vertebrae, hip, ischium, kidney, liver, shen men, sympathetic.

Diet

• Avoid cold, raw foods or iced drinks.

• Eat foods that tonify the qi and blood.

BURNS

Burns are generally classified according to their degree of severity:

FIRST-DEGREE BURNS: Most often occur because of sunburn. The skin is red, hot, and dry. If the sunburn is extensive, there may be fever.

SECOND-DEGREE BURNS: The skin is red and there are raised, fluid-filled blisters.

THIRD-DEGREE BURNS: There are blisters and ulcerations of the skin. The skin and the tissues under it are destroyed by the heat.

First Aid

1. The single best remedy for all three types of burns is Ching Wan Hung burn ointment. This product is available from Chinese pharmacies for a few dollars. It immediately relieves the pain and reduces blisters. It works effectively even for third-degree burns from hot steam and molten metal. Ching Wan Hung burn ointment contains ingredients that kill pain, reduce heat in the skin, and regenerate flesh.

    To use: Cover the burned area liberally with the ointment and then cover with a thin sterile gauze dressing.

    • For sunburn, there is no need to use the gauze.

    • For second-degree burns, do not pop the blisters. Apply the ointment thickly over the blisters and cover with gauze.

    • For third-degree burns, apply the ointment and see a doctor immediately.

    Any extensive burn or burns, particularly those that cause fever or vomiting or nausea, should be seen by a physician.

2. For sunburn, rub the burned areas with the inside of a watermelon rind.

Follow-up Treatment

1. Once the burn is healing, apply aloe and moisturizers to help with the dryness.

2. If there is scarring, a paste made of **pure pearl powder** (chapter 8) can help minimize the scarring and help the flesh regenerate.

Diet

During the healing process:

- avoid alcohol and hot, spicy foods.

- avoid deep-fried fatty foods.

- eat fruits and drink fruit juice to help bring moisture to the skin and flesh.

- eat more light foods and reduce the intake of heavy, rich foods.

- increase your intake of fluids.

CONCUSSION

Impact injuries to the head can bruise the brain and or cause it to bleed between the skull and the meninges (the membranes that form a wrapping around the brain). Pooled blood can create pressure on the brain. There may be loss of consciousness, blurry vision, and nausea. The head aches and one pupil is sometimes more dilated than the other. If there is bleeding, the headache can worsen steadily rather than improve over time.

First Aid

1. Go to a hospital or see your doctor immediately. If there is bleeding, this injury can be especially serious.

2. Elevate the head of the person slightly when he or she is lying down. Stabilize the head and neck to keep both immobile when the injured person is being transported.

3. Take **yunnan paiyao**—2 capfuls of powder or 3 capsules twice a day for several days, provided you are not vomiting (chapter 8); but still see a doctor.

4. Press the **P 6** acupoint to help relieve nausea (chapter 13).

Follow-up Treatment

1. Avoid getting another concussion for at least 6 months. Two or more concussions that occur with 6 months can make you susceptible to minor concussions triggered by even a slight impact to the head.

2. Press the **LI 4** acupoint frequently to relieve any residual headache (chapter 13).

Diet

Avoid spicy foods until well after the bleeding is stopped or the bruising is healed.

CONTUSIONS/BRUISES

Contusions are bruises. They can penetrate to the skin or down through the muscle to the bone, depending on the force of the impact that caused the injury. The force of the impact ruptures blood vessels beneath the skin. This black-and-blue spot that we call a bruise is actually a hematoma, a pooling of blood from broken vessels inside the muscles and tissues of the injured area. Tendons, ligaments, and even the periosteum, the outer lining of the bone, can be contused. Although minor contusions often get better on their own, it is best to treat all contusions as though they are serious. Improperly treated contusions can interfere with daily activities or sports performance for weeks or even months.

First Aid

1. Massage **trauma liniment** (chapter 11) into the injured area. If there is a lump, use the trauma liniment to rub over the lump, pressing gently to disperse accumulations of fluid and blood. If the contusion is more than just a minor bruise, follow this by wrapping the area in gauze and soaking it with trauma liniment.

2. Take two **trauma pills** a day for 2 days or take **Resinall K** twice a day for 2–3 days (chapter 15).

3. If the contusion is more severe and to a large muscle area such as the biceps or thigh, apply **san huang san** (chapter 11) mixed with egg whites to the discolored area.

Follow-up Treatment

1. If the bruise is felt but not seen and still sore after 2 or 3 days, the periosteum of the bone may be bruised. Apply **black ghost oil** (chapter 10) instead of trauma liniment.

2. Do gentle range-of-motion and stretching exercises.

Exercises

Once the initial inflammation is gone, do the **Daily Dozen** (chapter 5) and the **Eight Brocade Plus** (chapter 6) to restore strength and flexibility to the injured area.

Acupoints and Massage

Ear points: shen men, sympathetic, and the point relating to the area of the body injured.

Diet

- Avoid cold, raw foods and iced drinks.

CUTS, LACERATIONS, AND PUNCTURES

With any open wound, it is important to first stop the bleeding by direct pressure, then apply herbal remedies like **yunnan paiyao** (chapter 8). In small wounds or puncture wounds where there is no danger of excessive blood loss, let the wound bleed for a minute to clean out any dirt or bacteria that may have gotten inside. Next clean the wound thoroughly. Soap and water are the most effective means of cleaning wounds, followed by irrigation with hydrogen peroxide. Make sure any dirt, gravel, or splinters are removed from the wound. Any extensive loss of blood should be treated immediately by a physician. See chapter 8 for a more detailed discussion of treating open wounds.

First Aid

1. Stop the bleeding.

2. Clean the wound.

3. Apply yunnan paiyao as a powder until the bleeding stops. Take a capful of the powder or 2–3 capsules orally with water to prevent infection and help stop the bleeding.

4. Once the bleeding is stopped, mix yunnan paiyao with your own saliva to make a paste, cover the wound with the paste, and then apply a bandage. Clean and reapply the paste twice a day until the wound is healed.

5. If there are extensive lacerations, simply sprinkle yunnan paiyao powder over the area and cover with a dressing.

Follow-up Treatment

When the scar is still active (red and tender), make a paste with your saliva and **pure pearl powder** (chapter 8) and apply to the scar 2–3 times a day. Alternatively, the pearl powder can be mixed with lemon juice.

Diet

- Until the wound is closed, avoid spicy foods.

- Avoid fatty, deep-fried foods.

DISLOCATIONS

A complete dislocation occurs when two bones are displaced from their normal positions and are no longer in contact with each other. In a partial dislocation, the muscles, tendons, and ligaments are strong enough to hold the bones together, so they are forced out of position for a moment and then snap back into position again. Depending on the joint that is injured, they may go back into position or may be slightly out of position. Partial dislocations are also called "subluxations."

Dislocations are extremely painful until the bones are returned to normal alignment. This usually requires treatment by a doctor, and the sooner it can be done the better. The pain dissipates rapidly once the joint is returned to its normal position. The problem with dislocations and subluxations is that tendons and ligaments become overstretched and there may be damage to the cartilage or the joint itself. This predisposes the joint to being injured or dislocated again. The shoulder joint in particular is prone to repeat dislocations, which is why surgery is often recommended by doctors when there are repeated dislocations in this joint.

First Aid

Once the joint is back in place:

1. Apply **san huang san** (chapter 11) mixed with egg whites to reduce inflammation and swelling, or use **Wu Yang pain-relieving plaster** or **yunnan paiyao plaster** (chapter 11).

2. Take 1 **trauma pill** 2 times a day for 2 days, or take **Resinall K** for 2–3 days (chapter 15).

3. Massage acupoints that affect the injured area (see chapter 13). For example:

- For the shoulder, press **TH 3** on the opposite side of the body from the injury and **LI 10** on the side that is injured.

- For the wrist, press **LI 10** and **SI 11**.

- For the hip, press **ST 31** and **ST 36**.

4. Apply **trauma liniment** (chapter 10) to the injured area.

Follow-up Treatment

1. Apply **701 plasters** or **gou pi plaster** (chapter 11) to the injured area.

2. Apply **tendon lotion** (chapter 10) to the injured area several times a day.

3. Take **bone-knitting powder** (chapter 15) for 2–3 weeks to help the body repair the injured soft tissue.

4. Apply the **sinew-bone poultice** (chapter 11). Prepare by cooking the powder with alcohol and honey.

5. Heat the area with a moxa stick (chapter 16).

Exercises

Exercises are specific to the injured area and must be aimed at strengthening the muscles that support and stabilize the joint. For example, in the shoulder area it is important to strengthen the rotator cuff muscles. Initially avoid exercises that take the joint through a wide range of motion.

- **Shoulder:** See "Shoulder—Rotator Cuff Tear."

- **Wrist:** See "Wrist—Sprain/Strain."

- **Hip:**

    1. Sit in a chair with the feet flat on the floor and press outward against the resistance of your hands with your knees.

    2. Push for 10 seconds and relax for 10 seconds. Repeat 10 times—do this exercise 2–3 times a day.

    3. Do the **pillow squeeze exercise** (see "Knee—Pain under the Kneecap").

    4. When the hip gets stronger, progress to the **slow walk exercise** (see "Achilles' Tendonitis").

- **Knee:** See "Knee—Torn Ligaments."

- Finally, progress to the **Eight Brocade Plus** exercises (chapter 6).

Acupoints and Massage

1. Massage the injured area frequently to bring circulation to the area. It may be useful to use **black ghost oil** because of its ability to penetrate deeply into the joint.

2. **Ear points:** shen men, liver, kidney, sympathetic, point related to injured area.

Diet

- Eat foods that nourish the qi and blood.

- Introduce more sour foods into your diet, especially if they are also nourishing (for example, liver or Liquid Liver Extract, beef tendon, or beef cooked with vinegar).

- Avoid shellfish and cold foods or iced drinks.

ELBOW—TENNIS AND GOLFER'S

Both of these conditions involve an inflammation of the muscles and tendons of the forearm where they attach to the elbow. Tennis elbow is a strain of the extensor muscles, which attach to lateral epicondyle on the outer side of the elbow. Golfer's elbow is a strain of the flexor muscles, which attach to the medial epicondyle on the inside of the elbow. These injuries are the result of improper technique, usually using the wrist and elbow too much rather than the unified power of the legs, body, shoulder, and arm. Tennis elbow and golfer's elbow can also be caused or exacerbated by playing too hard, too frequently, without allowing sufficient time for the body to recuperate.

Tendonitis of the elbow is not exclusive to golfers and tennis players. It can happen to carpenters, mechanics, massage therapists, or anyone who repetitively uses the wrist and elbow to generate force. These injuries can be slow to heal for three primary reasons:

1. Tendons are thick fibrous tissues. Unlike muscle tissue, tendons do not have a large direct supply of blood to bring nutrients and fluids to damaged tissues. Therapies that encourage local circulation will help reduce healing time.

2. These injuries are the result of faulty body mechanics and improper technique. You must learn to use the arm properly. This may involve reeducation in the techniques specific to the sport as well as daily performance of exercises that reeducate the body and teach it to use the arms properly.

3. Athletes or busy people tend not to allow sufficient time for the body to rest after an injury.

First Aid

1. Apply **san huang san** (chapter 11) to the injured area. Alternatively, apply **Wu Yang pain-relieving plaster** or **yunnan paiyao plaster** (chapter 11).

2. Massage **trauma liniment** (chapter 10) gently into the tendons where they attach to the bone. Press only to the level of the tendon, not down to the bone. Use **circular pressing** toward the bone to apply the liniment.

3. Take **Resinall K** twice a day for 4–6 days (chapter 15).

Follow-up Treatment

1. Massage **tendon lotion** or **U-I oil** (chapter 10) gently into the tendons where they attach to the bones, several times a day.

2. Apply **701 Plasters** (chapter 11).

Exercises

1. Do the **Daily Dozen** (chapter 5), especially **Neck, Open and Close, Arm Rotation, Elbow Rotation, Pulling Nine Oxen,** and **Sinew Stretching.**

2. Do the **Eight Brocade Plus** (chapter 6), especially **Supporting the Sky with Both Hands, Drawing the Bow to Shoot the Eagle, The Black Dragon Enters the Cave,** and **Clenching the Fists and Glaring Increases Strength.**

3. Hold the tiger push posture while focusing on relaxed abdominal breathing. When assuming this posture, let the elbows fall inward slightly so there is a faint spreading sensation across the upper back. (Figure 136.)

Acupoints and Massage

1. Press **LI 4** and **LI 10** frequently throughout the day. For golfer's elbow, you may also press **P 6**.

2. **Grasp** the muscles of the forearm until they are relaxed, followed by **stroking** the arm from the elbow to the fingertips 10–20 times. Do this 2–3 times a day.

3. **Ear points:** elbow, sympathetic, shen men, liver, spleen.

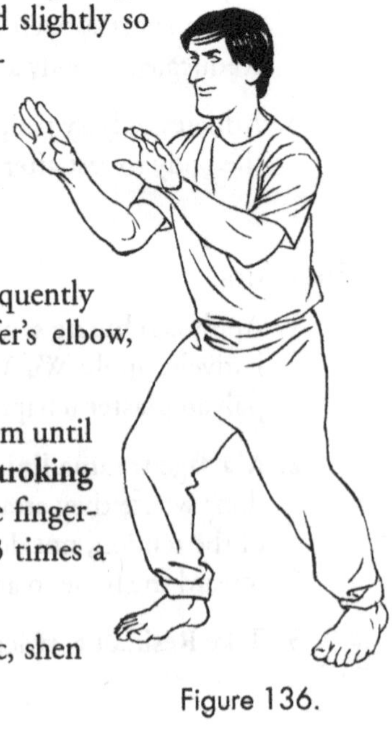

Figure 136.

Diet

- Avoid shellfish.

- Avoid cold foods and iced drinks.

- Avoid or reduce intake of sour foods.

EYE—CONTUSION (BLACK EYE)

Bruising around the eye from a blow that hits the bony structures that surround the eye is usually not a serious injury, unless the bones around the eye are also fractured. If there is a fracture, see "Fractures," using therapies appropriate to the site of the injury. Poultices, plasters, and most liniments cannot be used over or around the eye.

First Aid

1. Massage the swollen area with **trauma liniment** (chapter 10). Press gently on the swelling and then gently **thumb push** (see chapter 14) away from the eye. Avoid getting the liniment in the eye.

2. Take **Resinall K** (chapter 15) twice a day for 2 days. You can also massage the swollen area with it.

3. If the skin around the eye is cut and bleeding, take 1 capful of **yunnan paiyao** (chapter 8) or 2 capsules. Stop the bleeding with direct pressure. Make a paste of yunnan paiyao by mixing the powder with your saliva and apply thinly over the area. Avoid getting it in the eye.

Follow-up Treatment

If the skin around the eye was cut:

1. Apply a small piece of the membrane inside an eggshell over the wound. As it dries, it will draw the edges of the wound together. Leave it for several days. It will either fall off by itself or you can wet it with a damp cloth to make it come off (see chapter 8).

2. The wound should now be a closed thin red line. Once the wound is closed but the scar is still active—that is, it is still red and tender—apply **pure pearl powder** by making it into a paste with your saliva or mixing it with lemon juice (chapter 8). This will reduce scarring.

Diet

- **Bruising only:** Avoid cold, raw foods and drinks.

- **Bleeding:** Avoid spicy foods.

FINGER—JAMMED/SPRAINED

A jammed finger is a common minor injury that often goes untreated or is treated improperly. It is amazing how many people end up with crooked fingers that ache years later. A jammed finger is actually a subluxation (partial dislocation) of the joint. The bone is forced out of position and then snaps back into place again, usually in correct alignment, but not always. Because the tendency of the finger is to buckle to one side to protect the joint, the tendons on the side of the finger get twisted and damaged. It is often hard to completely reduce the swelling that occurs when a finger is badly jammed because the finger joints are encased in a tight joint capsule that traps stagnant fluids. Immediate treatment using a combination of complementary therapies and diligent follow-up treatment is often necessary to return the finger to normal.

First Aid

1. If the joint is swollen or black and blue, use a sterile lancet to bleed the swollen area.

2. Rub **trauma liniment** (chapter 10) into the finger, especially into areas of tenderness along the sides of the joint. Soak cotton balls with the liniment and tape over the swollen joint. This can be left on for up to 24 hours.

3. Take a **trauma pill** twice a day for 2–3 days. Alternatively, take **Resinall K** twice a day for 2–3 days (chapter 15).

4. Press **LI 4** and **LI 10** to relieve pain (chapter 13).

Follow-up Treatment

1. Massage **tendon lotion** or **U-I oil** into the injured area several times a day (chapter 10).

2. Apply **701 Plasters** (chapter 11) to the joint to prevent calcifications from forming.

3. Use the **tendon-relaxing soak** (chapter 12) 2 times a day for 7–10 days.

4. Heat the area with a moxa stick to reduce residual stiffness, pain, and swelling (chapter 16). Make sure you fumigate the joint in the smoke.

Exercises

1. Do the **Daily Dozen** (chapter 5), especially **Neck, Open and Close, Arm Rotation, Elbow Rotation, Pulling Nine Oxen,** and **Sinew Stretching.**

2. Do the **Eight Brocade Plus** (chapter 6), especially **Supporting the Sky with Both Hands, Drawing the Bow to Shoot the Eagle, Lift a Single Hand,** and **Black Dragon Enters the Cave.**

3. Practice the posture of holding a ball in front of the neck. (Figure 137.)

   Hold this posture for 2–5 minutes a day. Let the fingers spread so that the space be-

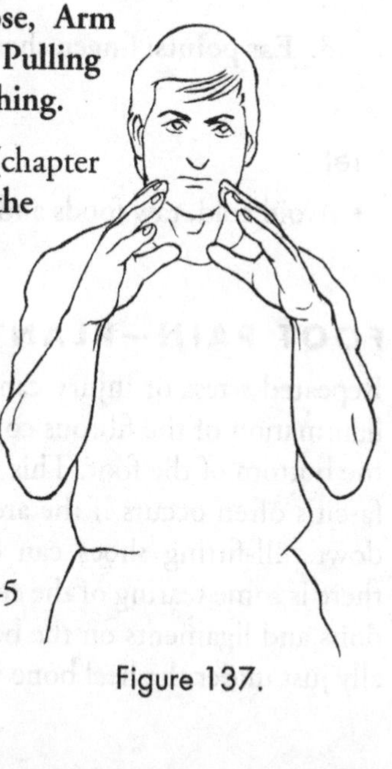

Figure 137.

tween the thumb and forefinger is open and relaxed and the center of the palm is slightly hollowed. Feel as though the fingertips and palm centers of the two hands are connected by a current of energy.

4. Practice rotating ba ding balls (Chinese steel balls that are solid or contain a chime inside) (Figure 138):

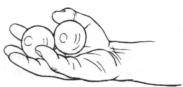

Figure 138.

- Rotate them in your hand so that the balls remain touching the whole time, rotating smoothly without any clacking sound.

- Rotate them smoothly so that the balls do not touch each other at all but circle smoothly in the hand.

Acupoints and Massage

1. Press **LI 4** and **LI 10** frequently throughout the day.

2. **Circular press** sore areas at the joint.

3. **Ear points:** finger, shen men, sympathetic, liver.

Diet

- Avoid cold, raw foods and iced drinks.

FOOT PAIN—PLANTAR FASCITIS

Repeated stress or injury can lead to chronic contraction and inflammation of the fibrous connective tissue (the plantar fascia) on the bottom of the foot. This is known as "plantar fascitis." Plantar fascitis often occurs if the arch is overstretched as the foot comes down. Ill-fitting shoes can contribute to the problem. Usually there is some tearing of the connective tissue and spasm of the tendons and ligaments on the bottom of the foot. The pain is generally just under the heel bone where the plantar fascia connects.

First Aid

Plantar fascitis usually develops over time, so that when it becomes a problem it is already chronic—a stage 2 or stage 3 sinew injury. If there is inflammation:

1. Apply **san huang san** (chapter 11) mixed with green tea to the inflamed area. Paint it on the area like a thin paste and wrap with gauze and an Ace bandage. It may be better to do this at night when you won't be putting your weight on the foot.

2. Apply **Wu Yang pain-relieving plaster** (chapter 11) to the underside of the heel.

Follow-up Treatment

1. Use the **tendon-relaxing soak** (chapter 12) twice a day.

2. Massage **tendon lotion** (chapter 10) into the painful area where the plantar fascia attaches to the heel, several times a day.

3. Apply **701 Plasters** (chapter 11) to the underside of the heel.

Exercises

1. Stretch the Achilles' tendon and the bottom of the foot by doing the **towel stretch** (see "Achilles' Tendonitis").

2. Roll a tennis ball on the bottom of the foot to massage and relax the plantar fascia. (Figure 139.)

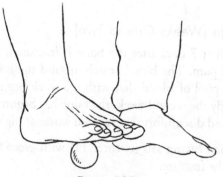

Figure 139.

Acupoints and Massage

1. Massage treatment:

   - **Press** and **circular press** acupoints **SP 4** and **KID 2**.

   - Then continue to press and circular press along that same line on the inside of the arch of the foot (between the bones and the muscles) until you reach the heel. **Grasp** and circular press around the sides of the heel.

   - Grasp and gently pluck the Achilles' tendon.

2. Rub **KID 1**—see exercise 18 of the **health preservation exercises** (chapter 7).

3. **Ear points:** heel, sympathetic, liver, kidney, shen men.

Diet

- Avoid shellfish.

- Reduce intake of sour foods.

- Avoid cold, raw foods and iced drinks.

FRACTURES

Treatment of fractures is discussed in detail in chapter 4. Chinese sports medicine divides fracture healing into three distinct stages.

Acute Stage (Weeks One to Two)

During the first 7 days after the bone is fractured, there is acute swelling and pain. The blood vessels around the bone also break and create a pool of blood that within a week begins to produce blood cells. By the second week, the bone has begun to knit, causing itching and discomfort that is often worse at night.

1. Mix **san huang san** (chapter 11) with green tea and apply over the fracture.

2. Apply **trauma liniment** (chapter 10) to the injured area gently by hand, or soak clothes in the liniment and apply like a poultice.

3. Take 1 **trauma pill** twice a day for 2–3 days or **Resinall K** twice a day for 2–4 days (chapter 15). If a rib is fractured, take the **rib fracture formula** instead (chapter 15).

4. Apply **Wu Yang pain-relieving plaster** or **yunnan paiyao plaster** (chapter 11) to the injured area.

5. Ear acupoints can be stimulated throughout the healing process in all 3 stages. **Ear acupoints:** shen men, sympathetic, kidney, liver, point that relates to the body area that is fractured (chapter 13).

Important: Liniments, poultices, and plasters cannot be applied in cases of compound or "open fractures" where the bone has penetrated the skin.

Knitting Stage (Weeks Three to Four)

This is a continuation of the end of the acute phase. The bones continue to knit as new bone is being formed. By the fourth week, the bones may have knit but are still soft and flexible at the site of the break.

1. If there is no infection, take **bone-knitting powder** (chapter 15) for 2–3 weeks, ¼ teaspoon 2 times a day.

2. Massage above and below the site of the fracture. Mainly use long, gentle stroking movements to encourage normal circulation and reabsorption of stagnant fluids.

3. Press acupoints that affect the fractured area several times a day (see chapter 13).

4. If possible, do isometric contractions of the muscles if the fracture is on one of the limbs.

Complete Healing (Weeks Five to Six)

In a simple complete ("clean") break, if the individual is healthy, the bones should be solid and strong by the end of the sixth week. More severe breaks may take longer, but correct treatment from the outset can greatly speed the healing process.

1. If the injured area is cold to the touch or aches in damp weather, apply the **sinew-bone poultice** (chapter 11).

2. If you did not take the **bone-knitting powder** (chapter 15) in the previous stage, take it at this stage to clear out residual stagnation and encourage the body to heal.

3. Massage above and below the site of the break and stimulate appropriate acupoints, as in the previous stages.

4. Use a moxa stick to heat the local area if all inflammation is gone and there is no infection (chapter 16).

Diet

- Avoid cold, raw foods and iced drinks.
- Eat foods that tonify the qi and blood.
- Avoid shellfish during the acute and knitting stages.
- Avoid fatty, fried foods.

GROIN MUSCLE—PULLED/STRAINED

Groin pulls involve a group of muscles known as the "adductors." The adductor muscles bring the legs together and stabilize the hip during walking, running, and pivoting movements. They can be injured through chronic overuse or by a sudden overstretching of the leg. They can also be injured through forced stretching. Groin pulls can be slow to heal and often recur unless they are treated properly. To prevent reinjury, the strength and flexibility of the adductors must be increased through exercises like the **Daily Dozen** (chapter 5) and the **Eight Brocade Plus** (chapter 6).

First Aid

1. Mix **san huang san** (chapter 11) with egg whites and apply to the local area. Wrap and leave on for 24 hours. Repeat applications of san huang san for up to three days if necessary. It may be necessary to apply san huang san thinly, as though "painting" it onto the muscle.

2. Massage **trauma liniment** (chapter 10) into the injured muscles, especially at their attachments at the groin. Avoid getting the liniment on the genitals.

3. Take 2 **trauma pills** a day for 2 days or **Resinall K** for 3–4 days after the injury (chapter 15).

4. Avoid ice, as it causes further contraction and stagnation. If you do use ice, apply for no more than 10–15 minutes per hour and only for the first 24 hours after the injury.

Follow-up Treatment

After pain, heat, and inflammation are gone or reduced, stretching and light exercise can be resumed with caution. Care must be taken to prevent reinjuring the muscle.

1. As you begin to stretch and strengthen the adductors (groin muscles), massage with liniments such as **U-I oil or Chinese Massage Oil** (chapter 10) before and after each exercise session. Avoid getting these liniments on the genitals.

2. Alternatively, when you are sure that heat (sensation of heat) and inflammation are gone, massage the area with **tendon lotion** (chapter 10).

3. Use the **tendon-relaxing soak** (chapter 12). Wet towels in the cooked herbs and apply to the injured hamstring for 10–15 minutes daily, especially after training. If you use this soak in combination with other liniments, lotion, poultices, and plasters, make sure you clean and dry the area before applying another lotion or poultice.

Exercises

1. Do the **Daily Dozen** (chapter 5), especially **Hula Hips and Hip Rotation, Knee Rotation, Phoenix Stretch,** and **Swing the Leg to Open the Hip.**

2. Do the **Eight Brocade Plus** (chapter 6), especially the **Leopard Crouches in the Grass** and **The Black Dragon Enters the Cave.**

3. Butterfly stretch: Sit on the floor with the soles of the feet together and the knees bent. Let the knees relax toward the floor. Use the palms to massage upward from the knees to the groin 15–20 times. This warms and relaxes the muscles and opens the meridians that run from the lower leg through the groin muscles. Then let the knees relax toward the floor with a sense of letting the hip open. Do not force the knees toward the floor. Do this exercise twice a day.

4. Massage the meridians of the legs—exercise 19 of the **health preservation exercises** (chapter 7).

5. Do the **slow walk exercise** (see "Achilles' Tendonitis").

Acupoints and Massage

1. Press **LIV 3** and **GB 34** to relax the muscles and tendons.

2. Massage treatment:

   • Gently **grasp** the groin muscles going from the knee to the groin.

   • **Palm push** the inner thigh muscles from the knee to the groin.

   • **Circular press** the areas of tenderness at the muscle attachments in the groin area.

3. **Ear points:** liver, shen men, external genitalia, sympathetic.

Diet

- Avoid or cut down on cold fluids, ice cream, and iced drinks.

- Avoid cooling, raw, or cold foods—raw vegetables and salads.

- Avoid or cut down on sour foods such as lemons, raw fruits, and fruit juices.

HAMSTRING—PULLED/TORN

A pulled hamstring is actually a torn muscle. This injury can be severe enough to bench a player for the entire season. Hamstring pulls often occur when an athlete fails to warm up properly. They are common among runners who run improperly dressed on cold, windy days. If a cold, contracted muscle is forced to stretch, it can easily tear. Forced stretching can cause a muscle pull, although it occurs more commonly with a sudden extension of the leg, as in kicking, or by a misstep in which the leg is forcefully extended. In these last two cases, the powerful quadriceps muscles in the front of the thigh contract, overstretching and tearing the hamstring. Often, an athlete is prone to a hamstring injury due to an imbalance in the muscles of the thigh. Trainers and physical therapists have known for years that the quadriceps should be only about 20 percent stronger than the hamstrings—a 60–40 ratio; yet athletes often overdevelop the quadriceps.

It is very common to reinjure a hamstring. This is usually a result of going back to play before the injury is fully healed and not taking the time to rehabilitate (strengthen and stretch) these muscles. Generally, a mild to moderate hamstring pull takes about 3 weeks to heal, while a severe pull may take as long as 6 weeks to heal completely.

Mild to Moderate Hamstring Pull

- Pain on stretching or extending the leg.

- Feeling of tightness on the injured side.

- Knots in the muscle.

- Hamstring muscle may feel swollen or inflamed.

- Discoloration or bruising in part of hamstring muscles.

Severe Pull

- Severe pain.

- Bunching up of muscle.

- Muscle weakness.

- Larger discoloration.

First Aid

1. Mix **san huang san** (chapter 11) with egg whites and apply to the local area. Wrap and leave on for 24 hours. Repeat applications of san huang san for up to 3 days if necessary.

2. Massage **trauma liniment** (chapter 10) into hamstring, going down back of leg and into space behind the knee.

3. Take 2 **trauma pills** a day for 2–3 days or **Resinall K** for up to 1 week after the injury (chapter 15).

4. Avoid ice, as it causes further contraction and stagnation. If you do use ice, apply for no more than 10–15 minutes per hour and only during the first 24–48 hours after the injury.

Follow-up Treatment

After pain, heat, and inflammation are gone or reduced, stretching and light exercise can be resumed with caution. Care must be taken to prevent reinjuring the muscle.

1. As you begin to stretch and strengthen the hamstrings, massage with liniments such as **U-I oil** or **Chinese Massage Oil** (chapter 10) before and after each exercise session.

2. Alternatively, when you are sure that heat (sensation of heat) and inflammation are gone, massage the area with **tendon lotion** (chapter 10).

3. If you can get someone to help you, lie on your stomach with a rolled towel under the thigh just above the knee. Have your friend massage the injured area with **tendon lotion** (chapter 10) by pressing into the muscle and stroking down toward the knee with one hand while the other hand gently pushes downward on the ankle, extending the leg and stretching the hamstring.

4. Use the **tendon-relaxing soak** (chapter 12). Wet towels in the cooked herbs and apply to the injured hamstring for 10–15 minutes daily, especially after training. If you use this soak in combination with other liniments, lotion, poultices, and plasters, make sure you clean and dry the area before applying another lotion or poultice.

Exercises

1. Increase flexibility of the hamstring muscles:

- Do the **Daily Dozen** (chapter 5) to enhance the body's flexibility and prevent reinjury. The **Phoenix Stretch** is particularly useful for hamstring injuries, because it not only stretches and relaxes the hamstring muscles, it also releases the lower back and sacrum. Often, it is tightness of the back and sacrum that causes a lack of flexibility in the hamstring, making it more prone to injury.

- Lie on the floor face-up with your legs propped up on the wall. This gently stretches the hamstrings and helps to release tension and holding in the lumbar area.

- Massage the meridians of the legs—exercise 19 of the **health preservation exercises** (chapter 7).

2. Increase the strength of the hamstrings:

- Do the **Eight Brocade Plus** (chapter 6) to strengthen the body in a balanced way. Of these, **Shake the Head and Wag the Tail, Squatting to Strengthen the Back and the Legs,** and **The Black Dragon Enters the Cave** are particularly useful.

- Leg curls: Using an ankle weight, lie on the stomach or support yourself on knees and elbows and bend the leg, pulling the heel toward the buttocks. Start with a light weight (a weight that allows you to do 15 repetitions without straining yourself) and slowly progress to a heavier weight. Do 3 sets of 5 repetitions every other day.

Acupoints and Massage

1. Tennis ball massage: Sit on the floor with your legs extended and the tennis ball under your thigh. Roll the ball up and down the back of the thigh by pushing the body forward and backward. Try to loosen up knots and stiff areas this way.

2. Massage treatment:

   - **Grasp** the back of the legs from the buttocks to the back of the knee.

   - **Palm push** from the buttocks to the back of the knee.

   - Use the fingertips to **circular press** the areas of tenderness under the buttock and behind the knee.

3. **Ear points:** shen men liver spleen, buttock, lumbar vertebrae, ischium.

Diet

- Avoid or cut down on cooling foods, such as raw juices, raw vegetables, salads, and the like, while the injury is healing.

- Avoid drinking cold fluids and or iced drinks. Try to have beverages at room temperature.

- Avoid sour foods.

HEEL SPUR

A heel spur is a hard, bony shelf or projection of the calcaneus (heel bone), caused by repeated pulling on the plantar fascia—the muscles and fibrous tissues on the underside of the foot that run from the heel to the metatarsal bones at the base of the toes. Repeated stress or injury can lead to chronic contraction and inflammation of the tendons and ligaments that make up the plantar fascia. Often, it occurs if the arch is overstretched as the foot comes down. This is known as "plantar fascitis." When plantar fascitis becomes chronic, the constant inflammation can cause calcium to be deposited on the bottom of the heel, forming a projection or spur. Spurs can also be formed by the plantar fascia pulling the periosteum (the fibrous membrane covering the bones) away from the bone, forming a bony projection that is painful when stepped on.

The main symptom is a deep discomfort under the heel when walking, running, or engaging in other weight-bearing activities. There may also be redness or a feeling of heat in the area. Sometimes the bony projection can be easily felt with the fingers.

Heel spurs usually form on the bottom of the heel but can also develop from repeated inflammation of the Achilles' tendon (Achilles' tendonitis). In this case, calcification and bone spurs can develop higher on the heel at the attachment of the Achilles' tendon.

First Aid

1. Use **san huang san** (chapter 11) when there is severe inflammation or redness in the area. It is particularly useful during the inflammatory stage before the spur forms (see "Foot Pain—Plantar Fascitis" and "Achilles' Tendonitis"). Use green tea as a medium to mix san huang san, as its cooling properties work to help reduce inflammation.

2. **Wu Yang pain-relieving plaster** (chapter 11) can be used as an alternative to san huang san.

3. Put doughnut- or horseshoe-shaped pads in the shoes that protect the spur from pressure to help reduce further irritation.

Follow-up Treatment

1. **The 701 Plasters** (chapter 11) help bring circulation to the area and can actually reduce the spur. As these plasters are somewhat warming, they must be used carefully or not at all if there is visible redness or a feeling of heat in the area.

2. Take **osteophyte powder** (chapter 15), ¼ teaspoon twice a day, for several months.

3. Soak the foot in **tendon-relaxing soak** (chapter 12) twice a day, followed by stretching and massaging the area. Clean your foot thoroughly after soaking, and allow some time to pass before applying other liniments or lotions.

Exercises

1. Gently stretch the muscles on the bottom of the foot by pulling back on the toes, or do the **towel stretch** (see "Achilles Tendonitis").

2. Do the **Daily Dozen** (chapter 5), especially the **Phoenix Stretch** and **Knee Rotation**.

3. Progress to the **slow walk exercise** (see "Achilles' Tendonitis").

Acupoints and Massage

1. Massage the **heel pain** acupoint on the hand opposite the painful heel.

2. Massage with fingers and thumbs around the painful area and then in long strokes along the bottom of the foot toward the toes. **Tendon lotion** or **U-I oil** (chapter 10) may be used for this purpose, or just use a light vegetable oil to reduce friction.

3. While seated in a chair, roll a tennis ball along the bottom of the foot. Avoid putting pressure on the spur.

4. **Ear points:** shen men, kidney, liver, heel.

Diet

- Take calcium with magnesium to balance the intake of the calcium. Cut down on calcium intake if you are taking large amounts; excessive calcium intake can lead to the formation of calcium deposits. The recommended amount of calcium per day is 1,200–1,500 mg with an equal amount of magnesium.

- Avoid drinking cold fluids and or iced drinks. Try to have beverages at room temperature.

- Avoid cold, raw foods.

HIP PAIN

Hip pain can have many origins. It can be referred from the low back area and wrap around the front of the hip. It can be the result of wearing of the cartilage that lines the articular surfaces of the ball-and-socket joint itself. Hip pain can be due to inflammation of the bursa, small, fluid-filled sacs that act to cushion joint structures and prevent rubbing and wear and tear. If a bursa becomes inflamed, pain and weakness can result. Impact injuries to the hip can damage the nerves that run over the prominence of bone in the front of the hip. This kind of injury is sometimes referred to as a "hip pointer." Additionally, the gluteal muscles and many of the thigh muscles cross in front of or behind the hip joint to attach to the femur. These muscles are susceptible to injury, misuse, and overuse.

First Aid

Liniments and poultices are not as effective in the hip area. The hip is hard to wrap and is surrounded by thick muscles, which make it hard for liniments to penetrate deeply enough.

1. If there is inflammation, apply **Wu Yang pain-relieving plaster** (chapter 11).

2. Alternatively, apply **701 plasters** or **yunnan paiyao plaster** (chapter 11).

3. If the hip aches in the cold, use **hua tuo anticontusion rheumatism plaster** (chapter 11).

4. Cup tender areas of the hip or buttocks (chapter 9).

5. Massage **trauma liniment** (chapter 10) into sore areas.

Follow-up Treatment

1. Soak towels in the **tendon-relaxing soak** (chapter 12) and apply them to the hip.

2. If pain is worse in cold weather, use the **warming soak** (chapter 12).

3. If pain is deep in the hip, rub **black ghost oil** (chapter 10) into tender areas.

Exercises

1. Do the **Daily Dozen** (chapter 5), especially **Hula Hips and Hip Rotation, Knee Rotation, Phoenix Stretch,** and **Swing the Leg to Open the Hip.**

2. Do the **Eight Brocade Plus** (Chapter 6), especially **Shake the Head and Wag the Tail, Squatting to Strengthen the Back and Legs,** and **The Leopard Crouches in the Grass.**

3. Standing with the feet shoulder width apart, roll the weight onto the inside edge of the feet and then roll the weight to the outside edge of the feet. Initiate these movements from the hips. Repeat 10–20 times. (Figures 140 and 141.)

4. Do the **slow walk exercise** (see "Achilles' Tendonitis").

5. Massage the meridians of the legs—exercise 19 of the **health preservation exercises** (chapter 7).

Acupoints and Massage

1. Press **ST 31, ST 36, GB 34,** and **GB 39.**

2. With the palms, rub in circles around the sacrum until it is warm, then continue rubbing in circles, moving around the sides of the hips to the front of the hips.

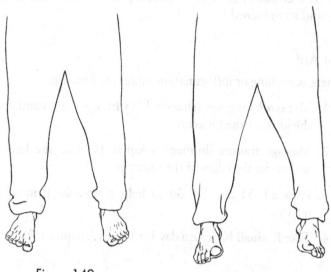

Figure 140.   Figure 141.

Diet

- Avoid or cut down on cooling foods, such as raw juices, raw vegetables, salads, and the like, while the injury is healing.

- Avoid drinking cold fluids and or iced drinks. Try to have beverages at room temperature.

KNEE—PAIN UNDER THE KNEECAP (Chondromalacia and Runner's Knee)

Chondromalacia and runner's knee often develop over time, with no specific injury as the culprit. Chondromalacia refers to a softening or wearing of the cartilage on the back of the kneecap. Runner's knee is caused by misalignment of the kneecap due to improper running or walking. Excessive pronation (an inward roll of the foot that causes the knee to rotate inward) causes the kneecap to track incorrectly in bending and extending movements. It rubs against the femur, gradually wearing down the cartilage. In both of these conditions, there is pain under the kneecap and there may be a creaking, grating, or popping sound when the knee is bent and straightened.

First Aid

If there is swelling or inflammation under the kneecap:

1. Mix **san huang san** (chapter 11) with egg whites and apply thickly over the kneecap.

2. Massage **trauma liniment** (chapter 10) into the kneecap and under the edges of the kneecap.

3. Press **ST 31** and **ST 36** to help relieve the pain (chapter 13).

4. Take **Resinall K** twice a day for 1 week (chapter 15).

Follow-up Treatment

1. Massage **tendon lotion** (chapter 10) into the kneecap and under the sides of the kneecap.

2. Use a moxa pole (chapter 16) to stimulate **ST 36** (chapter 13) and to heat up the knee. Follow this by massaging **U-I oil** (chapter 10) into the knee.

3. Apply the **sinew-bone poultice** (chapter 11) to the knee. Cover the kneecap completely.

4. Soak towels in the **warming soak** (chapter 12) and apply them to the knee for 15 minutes twice a day.

Exercises

1. Do the **Daily Dozen** (chapter 5), especially **Knee Rotation, Hula Hips and Hip Rotation,** and **Phoenix Stretch.**

2. Do the **Eight Brocade Plus** (chapter 6).

3. Do the **pillow squeeze exercise:** Stand and look in the mirror. The knees should be in line with the ridge of the shinbone.

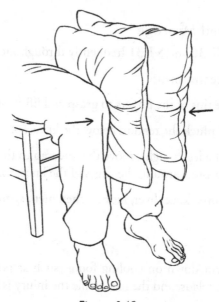

Figure 142.

- If the knees fall outward relative to the shinbone: Sit in a chair with your feet flat on the floor, thighs in line with your hips. The bend in the hip and the bend at the knee should be 90 degrees. The knees should be directly over the feet. Fill the space between the knees with firm pillows. Squeeze inward for 10 seconds. Pause and relax. Do 2–3 sets of 15 repetitions each twice a day. (Figure 142.)

- If the knees fall inward relative to the shinbone: Take the same position as above. Put your hands on the outside of the knees and push outward against your hands with the knees. Resist with your arms. Press outward for 10 seconds. Pause and relax. Do 2–3 sets of 15 repetitions each twice a day.

4. Do the **slow walk exercise** (see "Achilles' Tendonitis").

5. Massage the meridians of the legs—exercise 19 of the **health preservation exercises** (chapter 7).

Acupoints and Massage

1. Press **ST 36** and **ST 31** frequently throughout the day.

2. Massage treatment:

   • Use the tips of the fingers to **grasp** and lift the patella.

   • Gently **pluck** the tendon below the kneecap.

   • With the leg straight, move the kneecap to the side and **circular press** around the edges of the kneecap.

3. **Ear points:** knee, liver, kidney, shen men, sympathetic.

Diet

   • Avoid or cut down on cooling foods, such as raw juices, raw vegetables, salads, and the like, while the injury is healing.

   • Avoid drinking cold fluids or iced drinks. Try to have beverages at room temperature.

KNEE—TORN LIGAMENT
(Torn ACL or Medial Collateral Ligament)

The ligaments of the knee connect bone to bone. The medial collateral ligament stabilizes the inside of the knee, connecting the femur (thigh bone) to the tibia (shinbone). The lateral collateral ligament stabilizes the outside of the knee, connecting the femur to both the fibula and tibia. The anterior cruciate ligament (ACL) is inside the knee joint. It is a very strong ligament that prevents excessive front-to-back motion of the femur and tibia. If the force exerted by the athlete or the force of a blow to the knee is too strong, the bones pull apart, tearing the ligament.

The medial collateral ligament is injured more often than the lateral collateral ligament because blows or impacts to the outside of the knee are more common. Such an impact makes the knee fall inward, tearing the ligament. This is a common scenario in sports like skiing. A torn ACL can also be the result of an impact to the side of the knee. If it tears completely, you may hear a popping sound, after which the knee swells with blood. Partial tears of these structures can heal if treated properly—complete tears will not, but many people do fine with complete tears of the ACL, particularly if their leg muscles are strong. Unless you are playing sports like tennis, basketball, soccer, or football, all of which require sudden pivots and changes of direction, you may not need surgical repair of these ligaments. Reducing the swelling and strengthening the leg muscles around the knee can provide sufficient stability. Each case is different, and a lot depends on the stability of the joint and whether other structures were damaged as well. If the ACL, medial collateral ligament, and meniscus (cartilage) were all injured, the knee may be slow to heal or require surgical intervention.

First Aid

1. Apply **san huang san** (chapter 11) mixed with green tea to the entire knee area or the side of the knee that is injured. It may take 2–3 applications to bring down the swelling.

2. Take 2 **trauma pills** a day for 2–3 days. Alternatively, take **Resinall K** for 2–4 days twice a day (chapter 15).

3. Cup and bleed the swollen area (chapter 9).

4. Massage **trauma liniment** (chapter 10) into the knee. Massage above and below the swelling and then work the liniment gently into the swollen area.

5. Apply **yunnan paiyao plasters** (chapter 11) to swollen areas.

6. Press **ST 31, ST 36,** and **GB 34** to help relieve pain and reduce swelling (chapter 13).

Follow-up Treatment

1. Massage with **trauma liniment** (chapter 10) directly over the site of the injury. Push with the palm and the thumb from the injured area up the leg and from below the injured

area to the tips of the toes. This helps stagnant fluids and blood to be reabsorbed.

2. Use a moxa pole (chapter 16) to heat the knee and to stimulate **ST 36** (chapter 13).

3. Once the swelling, and redness are completely gone, mix the **sinew-bone poultice** (chapter 11) with honey and alcohol and apply to the knee. Apply 3 days in a row, stop for a day, and repeat for another 3 days. If the skin does not become irritated, this can be repeated for another week.

4. Take **bone-knitting powder** (chapter 15) for 2–3 weeks to help the body strengthen and repair damaged tissues.

Exercises

Slowly strengthen the knee and leg muscles by progressively moving through three stages of intensity.

Stage 1—when swelling subsides (acute):

- With the leg straight, tense the thigh muscles for 5 seconds and then relax. Do 3 sets of 20–30 repetitions several times a day.

- Sit with the leg straight. Put your palms on either side of the knee joint. Use your hands and arms to bend and straighten the knee, slowly but gently trying to increase the range of motion. Do this 10 times several times a day. Stimulating ear points (chapter 13) can help when doing this exercise.

- **Pillow squeeze exercise:** Sit in a chair with your feet flat on the floor, thighs in line with your hips. The bend in the hip and the bend at the knee should be 90 degrees. The knees should be directly over the feet. Fill the space between the knees with firm pillows. Squeeze inward for 10 seconds. Pause and relax. Do 2–3 sets of 15 repetitions each 3–4 times a day (see "Knee—Pain Under the Kneecap").

- Massage the meridians of the legs—exercise 19 of the **health preservation exercises** (chapter 7).

Stage 2—when you can straighten and bend the leg and you can support your weight on it.

- Hold the horse-riding posture. (Figure 143.) Make sure the knees are directly over the feet. The knee should not go past the kneecaps. Feel the weight settle into the whole foot evenly and let the tailbone sink under and keep the head erect with the tongue on the roof of the mouth.

- Leg extension exercise: Sit in a chair or on a bench or counter. Initially bend and extend the leg without resistance. (Figure 144.) Later add ankle weights, starting with as little as a pound. Gradually increase the weight. Eventually, the resistance should be enough so that in a set of 10–12 repetitions, the last repetition will be difficult to complete. Do 2 sets several times a day.

- Do the **slow walk exercise** (see "Achilles' Tendonitis").

Stage 3—when you can walk normally on stairs and hills.

Figure 143.

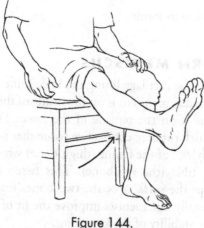

Figure 144.

- Do the **Daily Dozen** (chapter 5), especially **knee rotation, Hula Hips and Hip Rotation**, and **Phoenix Stretch.**

- Do the **Eight Brocade Plus** (chapter 6).

Acupoints and Massage

1. Frequently press **ST 36** and **GB 34** throughout the day.

2. Massage treatment:

- **Circular press** with the thumbs and the palms on the sides of the knee.

- **Press** the "eyes of the knee" (the depressions below the kneecap).

3. **Ear points:** knee, shen men, sympathetic, kidney, liver.

Diet

- Avoid or cut down on cooling foods, such as raw juices, raw vegetables, salads, and the like, while the injury is healing.

- Avoid drinking cold fluids and or iced drinks. Try to have beverages at room temperature.

- Avoid or cut down on shellfish.

- Cut down on sour foods.

KNEE—TORN MENISCUS

The meniscus is the cartilage lining the knee joint. There are two menisci. The medial meniscus is on the inside of the knee, and the lateral meniscus is on the outside of the knee. The menisci are composed of thick rubbery connective tissue that pads the projections, or "condyles," of the femur (thigh bone) where they fit into grooves in the tibia (the shinbone). This tissue is smooth and glossy and keeps the surfaces of the two bones from rubbing together. Additionally, the menisci improve the fit of the two bones and increase the stability of the knee joint.

The meniscus is usually injured by a twisting movement of the knee when the foot is planted on the ground. This can be the result of a sudden pivot or turn or an impact to the side of the knee, as in a football tackle. In these situations, the femur may pinch or grind down on the meniscus, tearing it. Usually the knee will swell and become hard to bend. If the lateral meniscus is torn, there will often be more pain on the outside of the knee. If the medial meniscus is damaged, there is usually more pain on the inside of the knee. A torn meniscus can weaken the stability of the knee joint and allow movement within the joint, which further grinds and tears the cartilage. If the tear is serious, it may require surgery, but in many cases surgery is not required.

First Aid

1. Apply **san huang san** (chapter 11) mixed with green tea to the entire knee area or the side of the knee that is injured. It may take 2–3 applications to bring down the swelling.

2. Take 2 **trauma pills** a day for 2–3 days. Alternatively, take **Resinall K** for 2–4 days twice a day (chapter 15).

3. Cup and bleed the swollen area (chapter 9).

4. Massage **trauma liniment** (chapter 10) into the knee. Massage above and below the swelling and then work the liniment gently into the swollen area.

5. Apply **yunnan paiyao plaster** (chapter 11) to swollen areas.

6. Press **ST 31**, **ST 36**, and **GB 34** to help relieve pain and reduce swelling (chapter 13).

Follow-up Treatment

1. Massage with **trauma liniment** (chapter 10) directly over the site of the injury. Push with the palm and the thumb from the injured area up the leg and from below the injured area to the tips of the toes. This helps stagnant fluids and blood to be reabsorbed.

2. Use a moxa pole (chapter 16) to heat the knee and to stimulate **ST 36** (chapter 13).

3. Once the swelling and redness are completely gone, mix the **sinew-bone poultice** (chapter 11) with honey and alcohol and apply to the knee. Apply 3 days in a row, stop for a day, and repeat for another 3 days. If the skin does not become irritated, this can be repeated for another week.

4. Take **bone-knitting powder** (chapter 15) for 2–3 weeks to help the body strengthen and repair damaged tissues.

Exercises

See "Knee—Torn Ligaments."

Acupoints and Massage

1. Frequently press **ST 36** and **GB 34**.

2. Massage treatment:

   • **Circular press** with the thumbs and the palms on the sides of the knee.

   • **Press** the "eyes of the knee" (the depressions below the kneecap).

3. **Ear points:** knee, shen men, sympathetic, kidney, liver.

Diet

• Avoid or cut down on cooling foods, such as raw juices, raw vegetables, salads and the like, while the injury is healing.

• Avoid drinking cold fluids and or iced drinks. Try to have beverages at room temperature.

• Avoid or cut down on shellfish.

• Cut down on sour foods.

- Take Liquid Liver Extract, a product available at many health food stores. Eating liver helps to strengthen the liver and thereby repair damaged tendons, ligaments, and cartilage.

MUSCLE CRAMPS/SPASMS

Muscle cramps do not have a single cause. A sudden muscle cramp can be the result of a number of factors:

- Not warming up properly, especially in cold weather.

- Overworking a muscle or group of muscles.

- Salt depletion from overexertion in hot weather.

- Sudden overstretching of a muscle.

- A slight tear in the muscle.

Cramps or muscle spasms that occur more chronically are usually the result of a systemic imbalance or improper use of the muscles around a joint. For example, chronic cramps of the feet and calf can be the result of a calcium deficiency. In this case, taking calcium with magnesium will quickly correct this problem. In Chinese medicine, however, chronic spasms can also be the result of a deficiency of blood. If the blood does not adequately nourish the tendons with blood, they spasm. This is analogous to a car engine that runs out of oil, resulting in the engine seizing. If there is a blood deficiency, dietary modifications may be necessary as well as treatment with acupuncture and herbs from a licensed practitioner of traditional Chinese medicine.

Other causes of muscle spasms can be diabetes or liver disease. A number of medications can also cause muscle spasms, so check the side effects of any medications you are on if you are experiencing chronic cramping.

First Aid

1. Press **GB 34** and **LIV 3** to relax the liver and ease the spasms (chapter 13).

2. Massage the muscle or muscles that are in spasm. If possible, use **U-I oil** or **Chinese Massage Oil** (chapter 10) as a massage oil, as these two liniments penetrate muscle tissue to improve circulation of energy and blood.

3. Do relaxed abdominal breathing.

Follow-up Treatment and Prevention

1. Warm up properly before beginning exercise or sports activities.

2. Massage **U-I oil** or **Chinese Massage Oil** (chapter 10) into the muscles before and after exercise and sports.

3. Make sure you are not suffering from a calcium deficiency. If you are, take calcium with magnesium.

4. Do the **Daily Dozen** (chapter 5) and the **Eight Brocade Plus** (chapter 6) to teach muscles to contract and relax at the proper times.

Acupoints

1. Frequently press **LIV 3** and **GB 34**.

2. Ear points: liver, shen men, sympathetic, point relating to body area that is in spasm or spasms chronically.

Diet

• Avoid or cut down on cooling foods, such as raw juices, raw vegetables, salads, and the like.

• Avoid drinking cold fluids and or iced drinks. Try to have beverages at room temperature.

• Cut down on sour foods.

NECK STRAIN/SPRAIN

Neck strains result when one or more muscles or tendons in the neck are overstretched through improper use or overuse. Alternatively, a sudden overstretching of the muscles and tendons can also cause a strain. Neck sprains occur when a ligament is overstretched. Because ligaments connect bone to bone, sprains usually occur when a violent force overstretches the neck, pulling one or more vertebrae out of their normal location. A classic example is a whiplash injury, in which the joints of the neck are pulled out of place and then snap back into position. The ligaments can become overstretched, making the joint unstable. Whiplash injuries, whether they occur in a car or on the football field, can cause compression or rupture of cervical discs or damage to the spinal cord and should be examined as soon as possible by a medical professional.

In both a neck strain or a neck sprain, there is usually some overstretching and tearing of tissue, which causes the muscles and tendons in the area to go into spasm. There may be some swelling and weakness in the area, and the neck will be stiff and sore. In some cases, it may be impossible to turn one's head. With a sprain, the pain may be more severe and there may be visible bruising as well. If there is disc impingement, there may be numbness or tingling down the arm. Keep in mind, however, that numbness and tingling can also be caused by tight muscles in the shoulders or neck that press on nerves. The presence of a herniated disc does not automatically explain referred pain or numbness.

Strained muscles generally heal quickly, especially if tears are small. A sprained neck takes longer to heal, as long as six weeks. It may take longer if treated improperly. An additional consideration is that Chinese medicine views the neck as being particularly prone to wind and cold penetration. One cause of strained neck in Chinese medicine is sleeping in a draft or in front of a fan or air conditioner. This cold wind in contact with the neck can cause a stiff neck that is quite painful and must be treated with heat for the muscle spasm to relax. When your neck is injured, it helps to keep it warm at all times, even to the point of wearing a scarf when indoors in air-conditioning. This can greatly reduce healing time.

First Aid

1. Massage **trauma liniment** (chapter 10) into the sore area of the neck.

2. Cup the injured area (chapter 9). Never cup the front of the neck, however; only the large muscles on the back of the neck can be cupped.

3. Take 2 **trauma pills** a day for 2–3 days or **Resinall K** (chapter 15) twice a day for 2–4 days.

4. Apply **Wu Yang pain-relieving plaster** or **yunnan paiyao plaster** (chapter 11) to the injured area.

5. Press the **luo zhen,** the stiff neck point on the hand (chapter 13). Press the point that is on the opposite side of the body from the neck pain. For example, if pain is on the right side of the neck, use the luo zhen point on the left hand. While pressing the point, slowly and gently move and rotate your neck.

Follow-up Treatment

1. Soak towels in the **tendon-relaxing soak** (chapter 12) and apply them to the neck.

2. Soak a cloth or paper towel in **U-I oil** (chapter 10). Place the cloth over the injured area and apply wet heat in the form of hot towels or a hydroculator pack.

3. Massage **tendon lotion** (chapter 10) into the injured area several times a day.

4. In case of a neck sprain with damaged ligaments, take **bone-knitting powder** (chapter 15) for 2–3 weeks.

Exercises

1. Do the **Daily Dozen** (chapter 5), especially **Neck Exercise.** This is probably the most important exercise for neck injuries. Also do **Arm Rotation** and **Elbow Rotation.**

2. Do the **Eight Brocade Plus** (chapter 6), especially **Looking Backward and Twisting Like a Dragon** and **Embracing the Moon.**

3. Do the **health preservation exercises** (chapter 7), especially numbers 1–11.

Acupoints and Massage

1. Press **luo zhen** frequently throughout the day, as explained in the first-aid treatment. The acupoints **TH 3** and **GB 39** may also be pressed frequently for neck pain.

2. Press **LIV 3** and **GB 34** to relieve muscle spasms and to help stimulate healing of muscles and tendons.

3. With your thumb, **press** and **circular press** from the base of the skull down the muscles of the neck.

4. **Ear points:** cervical vertebrae, shen men, sympathetic, liver.

Diet

• Avoid or cut down on cooling foods, such as raw juices, raw vegetables, salads, and the like.

• Avoid drinking cold fluids or iced drinks. Try to have beverages at room temperature.

• Cut down on sour foods.

NOSEBLEED

Nosebleeds are a fairly common sports injury. Usually, nosebleeds are minor injuries in which the bleeding stops fairly quickly. Frequent nosebleeds can also be caused by internal imbalances. These kinds of nosebleeds require treatment from a licensed practitioner of traditional Chinese medicine to address the source of the problem, but the first-aid techniques described here will usually stop the bleeding. Although **yunnan paiyao** (chapter 8) is very effective for stopping bleeding due to trauma, it should not be used for chronic nosebleeds, which are often due to internal imbalances. If a nosebleed from a hard blow does not stop bleeding and is accompanied by dark, thick blood, you should see a doctor, as there may be damage to structures behind the cartilage of the nose. If the nose is flattened or crooked, it should be reset as soon as possible.

First Aid

1. Use a string or shoelace to stimulate acupoints of the hand (see chapter 8). This will often stop a nosebleed.

2. Pull the hair on the nape of the neck.

3. Wrap a piece of thread tightly around the middle knuckle of the middle finger. Wrap the middle finger of the hand opposite the nostril that is bleeding. If both are bleeding, wrap the middle fingers of both hands.

4. Take a capful of **yunnan paiyao** powder or 2–3 capsules (chapter 8).

5. Stuff the nose with cotton, tilt the head back, and apply direct pressure by pinching the bridge of the nose.

6. If the above methods do not work, apply ice to the nose for several minutes to stop the bleeding.

Diet

- Avoid spicy foods for twenty-four hours after the bleeding has stopped.

PIRIFORMIS SYNDROME AND SCIATICA

The piriformis is a small muscle that lies beneath the gluteal muscles. It is instrumental in supporting the gluteal muscles in extending and rotating the hip. If the hamstrings or quadriceps muscles of the thigh are weak, the piriformis is called upon to support these muscles in bending and extending movements. The piriformis is often strained through overuse. This is usually the result of muscle imbalances in the leg, which force it to contract unnecessarily. When the piriformis goes into spasm, it can feel like a lump under the larger gluteal muscles. The sciatic nerve runs beneath the piriformis muscle. When the piriformis goes into spasm from overuse or improper use, it often presses on the sciatic nerve, causing pain that runs down the back or side of the leg. This sciatic pain is often misdiagnosed as coming from a disc herniation. Although herniation of discs in the lumbar spine can cause sciatic pain, in fact many people with bulging discs do not experience sciatica. Muscles in the hip and buttock area like the piriformis are often responsible.

First Aid

1. Take 2 **trauma pills** a day for 2–3 days, or take **Resinall K** for up to 1 week after the strain occurs (chapter 15).

2. Massage **trauma liniment** (chapter 10) into the tight muscles.

Follow-up Treatment

1. Massage **tendon lotion** (chapter 10) into the injured area.

2. Use the **tendon-relaxing soak** (chapter 12). Soak hot towels in the soak and apply to the buttock area twice a day.

3. Before and after flexibility exercises, apply **black ghost oil** (chapter 10) to the buttock and hip area.

Exercises

1. Do the **Daily Dozen** (chapter 5), especially **Hula Hips and Hip Rotation, Knee Rotation, Phoenix Stretch,** and **swing the Leg to Open the Hip.**

2. Do the **Eight Brocade Plus** (chapter 6), especially **Shake the Head and Wag the Tail, Squatting to Strengthen the Back and Legs,** and **The Leopard Crouches in the Grass.**

3. Do the **slow walk exercise** (see "Achilles' Tendonitis").

4. Massage the meridians of the legs—exercise 19 of the **health preservation exercises** (chapter 7).

5. Gently stretch the piriformis. To stretch the right piriformis:

   • Sit on the floor with the left leg stretched out straight in front of you. Cross the ankle of the right leg over the left knee. Gently pull the right leg toward your chest with both hands.

   • Lie on your back with the left leg straight and the right leg bent and crossed over the left. The sole of the right foot should be flat on the floor. With your right hand, pull the front of the right hip toward the floor while the left hand pulls the right knee toward the floor in the opposite direction.

6. Sleep on the side that is not painful, with a pillow between your knees to avoid putting an uncomfortable stretch on the piriformis while you are sleeping.

7. Avoid putting your wallet into the pocket on the affected side.

Acupoints and Massage

1. Press **LIV 3**, **GB 34**, and **GB 39** to help relieve the muscle spasm.

2. The piriformis is hard to massage yourself; lie down with the gluteal and piriformis muscles on top of a tennis ball. Gently move the tense area back and forth on the ball.

3. **Palm push** downward along the sacrum and buttocks.

4. **Ear points:** shen men, buttock, hip, liver, spleen, sympathetic.

Diet

- Avoid or cut down on cooling foods, such as raw juices, raw vegetables, salads, and the like, while the injury is healing.

- Avoid drinking cold fluids and or iced drinks. Try to have beverages at room temperature.

- Avoid sour foods.

POISONOUS BITES

Most insect bites are merely annoying and itchy and painful for a short time. However, spider bites and the stings of centipedes, scorpions, and even wasps can be damaging to muscle tissue and even the nervous system. Some spider bites, like those of the brown recluse or the black widow, can cause necrosis (death) of healthy tissue. In Chinese medicine, toxins from poisonous bites are thought to travel not only through the muscle tissue, but also along the meridian pathways. Because the meridians ultimately have connections with the internal organs, it is theoretically possible for these toxins to affect the functioning of the organs by damaging the meridian pathways. Therefore, it is imperative to draw out or neutralize the poison from these kinds of bites as quickly as possible.

First Aid

1. Cup over the bite to draw out the poison. Sometimes it is necessary to bleed the area with a lancet and then use the cup to draw out blood and the poison from the local area (chapter 9).

2. After cupping, use water and green clay to make a poultice. Cover the bite and the swollen area around it with the wet clay. Green clay is used in beauty salons to draw toxins or impurities out of the skin. As the clay dries, it will draw more of the poison out of the skin. Leave the clay on for 2–3 hours.

3. Take **yunnan paiyao** (chapter 8) orally with warm water. Take 1 capful of the powder or 2–3 capsules twice a day for several days.

4. After drawing the toxins with green clay, mix yunnan paiyao powder with your own saliva. Apply this mixture to the bite.

Diet

- Avoid spicy foods.

- Avoid consuming alcohol.

SHOULDER—BURSITIS

Bursitis of the shoulder is an inflammation of the subacromial bursa. Bursae are enclosed, fluid-filled sacs that prevent adjacent structures from rubbing against one another. This reduces friction and therefore wear and tear on those structures. In the shoulder, the subacromial bursa lies under the point of the shoulder, where the scapula (shoulder blade) and the collarbone meet. The bursa provides a cushion between these bones and the shoulder joint itself and protects the muscles of the rotator cuff from being pressed on by the collarbone and scapula.

Usually, the bursa becomes inflamed from an injury to the shoulder or as a result of a history of chronic shoulder injury. Untreated, it can lead to pain when lifting the arm and is often a precursor to frozen shoulder. Pain discourages you from moving the shoulder, and eventually range of motion becomes limited. For this reason, it is very important to maintain the range of motion in the shoulder after it has been injured, by doing exercises that maintain flexibility without irritating the inflamed bursa.

First Aid

1. Cup and bleed the shoulder (chapter 9), particularly the point of the shoulder.

2. Apply a thin coat of **san huang san** (chapter 11) mixed with green tea to the entire shoulder. Alternatively, apply **Wu Yang pain-relieving plaster** (chapter 11) to the painful area.

3. Take 2 **trauma pills** a day for 2–3 days or **Resinall K** twice a day for 2–4 days (chapter 15).

4. Massage **trauma liniment** (chapter 10) into the shoulder several times a day.

5. Press **TH 3** and **LI 10** (chapter 13) to relieve pain and regain range of motion in the shoulder.

Follow-up Treatment

1. Apply **701 plasters** or **gou pi plaster** (chapter 11) to the shoulder.

2. Frequently massage the shoulder with **tendon lotion** (chapter 10).

3. When all redness and heat are gone, use a moxa pole to warm the shoulder (chapter 16).

Exercises

1. Do the **Daily Dozen** (chapter 5), especially **Neck Exercise, Arm Rotation, Elbow Rotation,** and **Sinew Stretching.**

2. Do the **Eight Brocade Plus** (chapter 6), especially **Drawing the Bow to Shoot the Eagle.**

3. Meridian massage of the arms—exercise 11 of the **health preservation exercises** (chapter 7).

4. Covering palm exercises: Do these exercises slowly and carefully, without muscular tension. Keep the shoulders down and relaxed, and let the eyes follow the hand throughout.

Covering palm:

- Put your left hand on the lower back. Turn the waist to the right and swing the right arm with the palm up to the right, as you inhale. The eyes follow the hand. (Figure 145.)

- Finish inhaling as you begin to turn the waist to the left, letting the hand move overhead. (Figure 146.)

- Exhale and finish turning the waist to the left. Simultaneously, the hand and arm sink and press downward as though covering a large pot with a pot lid. (Figure 147.)

- Repeat 6–10 times. Then do 6–10 repetitions with the left arm.

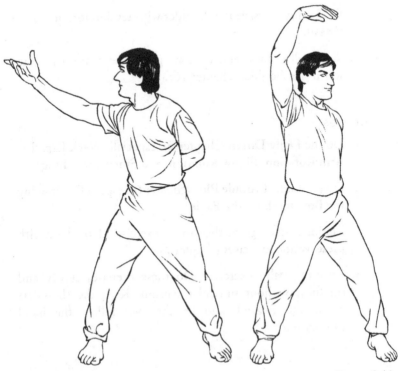

Figure 145.   Figure 146.

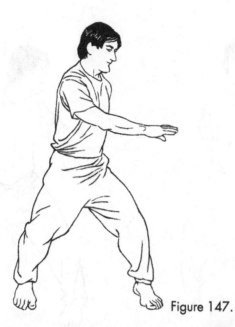

Figure 147.

Reverse covering palm:

- With the left hand on your lower back, inhale and turn the waist to the left, simultaneously letting the palm turn to face upward as you reach across the body with the right hand. Your eyes look at your right hand. (Figure 148.)

- Exhale as you begin to turn the waist to the right. The arm begins to turn as it rises overhead. The eyes follow the hand. (Figure 149.)

- Continue to exhale as the body finishes turning to the right. The hand and arm

Figure 148.

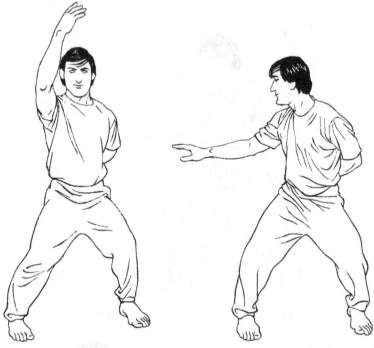

Figure 149.   Figure 150.

simultaneously sink downward as though covering a
large pot with a pot lid. (Figure 150.)

- Repeat 6–10 times. Then do 6–10 repetitions with the
  left arm.

Acupoints and Massage

1. Press **TH 3** on the side opposite the injured shoulder to relieve pain.

2. Press the **GB 39** on the side opposite the injured shoulder
   while moving and rotating the injured shoulder.

3. **Stroke** very lightly down the arm from the shoulder to the
   fingertips 10–12 times. Repeat this several times a day.

4. **Ear points:** shoulder, shen men, sympathetic, liver.

Diet

- Avoid shellfish.

- Avoid cold and raw foods and iced drinks.

- Avoid greasy, fatty foods.

SHOULDER—FROZEN SHOULDER

A frozen shoulder is not really a sports injury. It is the result of limiting the movement of the shoulder because you have injured it or because daily life does not require raising the arm or moving the shoulder through its full range of motion. The Chinese call frozen shoulder "fifty-year-old shoulder" because elderly and middle-aged people tend to be less active and are less inclined to use the full range of motion of the shoulder, particularly if they have injured the shoulder. Athletes who are active in sports on a daily basis rarely get frozen shoulder.

The best way to prevent frozen shoulder is to move your arm through its full range of motion every day, even if it is injured. Your frozen shoulder can move again. It requires patience and a willingness to move the arm even though it is painful. Eventually the muscles must also be strengthened. Exercises like the **Daily Dozen** (chapter 5) and the **Eight Brocade Plus** (chapter 6) were designed in part to prevent as well as rehabilitate this kind of problem.

Treatment

1. Apply **gou pi plaster** or **701 plasters** (chapter 11) to the shoulder joint.

2. If the shoulder is stiffer in cold weather or cold to the touch, use the **hua tuo anticontusion rheumatism plaster** (chapter 11).

3. Soak towels in the **tendon-relaxing soak** (chapter 12) and apply to the shoulder and shoulder blade to relax tight, spasmed muscles.

4. Apply **tendon lotion** (chapter 10) to the shoulder several times a day.

5. Cup the shoulder and shoulder blade (chapter 9). Then warm up the shoulder with a moxa stick (chapter 16).

Exercises

Begin with simple range-of-motion exercises:

1. Lift the arm and rotate it to face the chest and then lower the arm.

2. Bend over while holding a light weight and make circles with the arm. (Figure 151.)

3. Hold a bar or the branch of a tree and slowly lower the body by bending the knees. This is a good way to increase your ability to lift the arm. (Figure 152.)

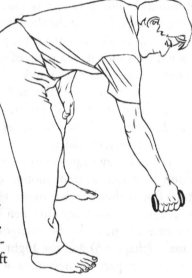

Figure 151.

4. Stand facing a wall and walk your fingers slowly up the wall. Then walk them up with your shoulder facing the wall.

5. Starting at the shoulder, use the palm of your other hand to pat up and down the arm from the shoulder to the fingertips. (Figure 153.)

6. Stand with arms shoulder level, palms facing downward. Exhale and throw the hands backward as though throwing something behind you. Inhale and let the arms recoil back to the start position. Repeat 20–30 times. (Figures 154 and 155.)

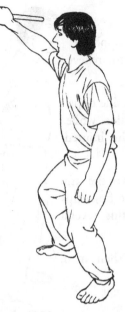

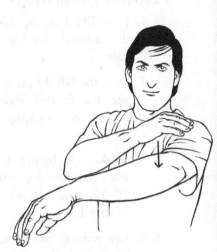

Figure 153.

Figure 152.

Start slowly and gently with a small range of motion and gradually increase amplitude, speed, and force. Keep the arms relaxed throughout.

As range of motion increases, add other exercises:

1. The **Daily Dozen** (chapter 5), especially **Neck Exercise, Arm Rotation, Elbow Rotation, Sinew Stretching, Slap Below the Nape,** and **Pulling Nine Oxen.**

2. The **Eight Brocade Plus** (chapter 6), especially **Supporting the Sky with Both Hands, Holding Up a Single Hand, Drawing the Bow to Shoot the Eagle,** and **Clenching the Fists and Glaring Increases Strength.**

3. The **covering palm exercises** (see "Shoulder—Bursitis").

Figure 154.

Acupoints and Massage

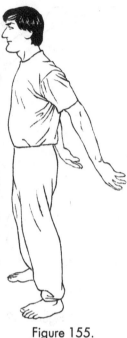

1. Press **TH 3** on the side opposite the injured shoulder to relieve pain.

2. Press the **GB 39** on the side opposite the injured shoulder while moving and rotating the injured shoulder.

3. **Stroke** very lightly down the arm from the shoulder to the fingertips 10–12 times. Repeat this several times a day.

4. **Ear points:** Shoulder, shen men, sympathetic, liver.

Diet

- Avoid shellfish.

- Avoid cold and raw foods and iced drinks.

- Avoid greasy, fatty foods.

- Cut down on sour foods.

Figure 155.

SHOULDER—ROTATOR CUFF TEAR

The rotator cuff is made up of four muscles: subscapularis, supraspinatus, infraspinatus, and teres minor. All four of these muscles attach to the scapula (shoulder blade) and the tubercles (bony projections) of the humerus (upper arm bone). The tendons of these four muscles form a cuff that helps to hold the joint together and control rotation of the shoulder. Overuse of the shoulder, particularly when the arm is overhead (as in pitching, tennis overhands and serves, and swimming), can cause a small tear in one or more of the rotator cuff muscles. Tearing of the rotator cuff can be caused by a single violent motion but is more often the result of wear and tear over time, particularly if the arm and shoulder are not being used correctly.

Usually, pain is felt in front of the shoulder where the rotator cuff is located. Sometimes a slight divot or depression in the muscle can be felt. With rotator cuff tears, as with all shoulder injuries, it is important to keep moving the arm to retain full range of motion and prevent frozen shoulder.

First Aid

1. Apply a thin coat of **san huang san** (chapter 11) mixed with green tea to the entire shoulder.

2. Alternatively, apply *Wu Yang pain-relieving plaster* or **yun-nan paiyao plaster** (chapter 11) to the painful area.

3. Take 2 **trauma pills** a day for 2–3 days or **Resinall K** twice a day for 2–4 days (chapter 15).

4. Massage **trauma liniment** (chapter 10) into the front of the shoulder several times a day.

5. Press **TH 3** and **LI 10** to relieve pain and regain range of motion in the shoulder.

Follow-up Treatment

1. Massage **tendon lotion** (chapter 10) into the front of the shoulder several times a day.

2. Apply **gou pi plaster** or **701 plasters** (chapter 11) to the injured area.

3. Heat the front of the shoulder with a moxa stick (chapter 16).

Exercises

1. Strengthen the rotator cuff using a light weight (from 1 to 3 pounds). Lay your arm over the edge of a chair or table, with the weight hanging down. (Figure 156.) The edge should contact the elbow crease. Raise the forearm to the

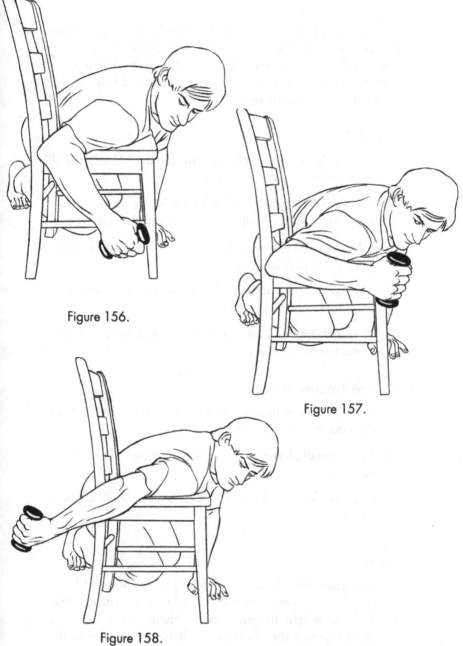

Figure 156.

Figure 157.

Figure 158.

front, then return to the neutral position. (Figure 157.) Repeat 10 times. Then raise the forearm to the back and return to the neutral position. (Figure 158.) Repeat this 10 times. This exercise isolates the rotator cuff.

2. Do the **Daily Dozen** (chapter 5), especially **Neck Exercise, Arm Rotation, Elbow Rotation, Sinew Stretching, Slap Below the Nape,** and **Pulling Nine Oxen.**

3. Do the **Eight Brocade Plus** (chapter 6), especially **Supporting the Sky with Both Hands, Holding Up a Single Hand, Drawing the Bow to Shoot the Eagle,** and **Clenching the Fists and Glaring Increases Strength.**

4. Do the **covering palm exercises** (see "Shoulder—Bursitis").

Acupoints and Massage

1. Press **TH 3** on the side opposite the injured shoulder to relieve pain.

2. Press the **GB 39** on the side opposite the injured shoulder while moving and rotating the injured shoulder.

3. **Stroke** very lightly down the arm from the shoulder to the fingertips 10–12 times. Repeat this several times a day.

4. **Ear points:** shoulder, shen men, sympathetic, liver.

Diet

• Avoid shellfish.

• Avoid cold and raw foods and iced drinks.

• Avoid greasy, fatty foods.

• Cut down on sour foods.

WRIST—SPRAIN/STRAIN

The wrist is a complex joint composed of eight small bones that articulate both with the radius and ulna (the bones of the forearm) and the bones of the hand (the metacarpals). Because of this complexity, it is subject to a variety of injuries. The impact from punching in sports like boxing and kickboxing can jam the metacarpal bones against the wrist bones, knocking them out of alignment. In racket sports like tennis, repeated impacts can injure the metacarpals and wrist bones, and the gripping motion can cause tendonitis where the tendons cross the wrist. The falls that are so common in snowboarding and in-line skating can also injure the wrist because the instinctive response is to extend your arm to break the fall. If the wrist is fractured, see also "Fractures." Otherwise, many of these injuries can be treated as a sprain or strain.

First Aid

1. Press **LI 10** and **LI 4** to relieve pain (chapter 13).

2. Massage **trauma liniment** (chapter 10) into the wrist and hand. If sprained, massage lightly over the swollen, black-and-blue area and more deeply above and below the sprain.

3. Mix **san huang san** (chapter 11) with green tea or Vaseline and apply to the wrist.

4. Take a **trauma pill** twice a day for 2–3 days. Alternatively, take **Resinall K** twice a day for 2–3 days (chapter 15).

5. If sprained, bleed and cup the area to reduce swelling and blood stagnation (chapter 9).

6. Perform simple range-of-motion exercises that do not aggravate the injury. If the sprain is severe, these may have to wait until there is less pain.

Follow-up Treatment

1. If the wrist was sprained, you can now massage with **trauma liniment** (chapter 10) directly over the site of the injury. Push with the palm and the thumb from the sprained area up the arm and from below the sprained area to the tips of the fingers. This helps stagnant fluids and blood to be reabsorbed.

2. Soak the wrist in the **tendon-relaxing soak** (chapter 12) to relax spasms in the tendons and muscles that are inhibiting range of motion.

3. If pain and stiffness are worse with the cold, massage **tendon lotion** or **U-I oil** (chapter 11) into the injured area.

4. Use a moxa stick to warm the area and help reduce any residual swelling (chapter 16). Moxa **LI 10** (chapter 13) and the wrist area.

Exercises

1. Do the **Daily Dozen** (chapter 5), especially **Arm Rotation, Elbow Rotation,** and **Pulling Nine Oxen.**

2. Do the **Eight Brocade Plus** (chapter 6), especially **Drawing the Bow to Shoot the Eagle, The Black Dragon Enters the Cave,** and **Embracing the Moon.**

3. Massage the meridians of the arms. Do exercise 11 of the **health preservation exercises** (chapter 7).

4. Practice the posture of holding a ball in front of the neck (see "Finger—Jammed").

5. Practice rotating the **ba ding balls** (See "Finger—Jammed").

Acupoints and Massage

1. Massage treatment:

   • **Grasp** the muscles of the forearm from the elbow to the wrist.

   • **Circular press** the tender areas of the wrist.

   • **Press LI 10** and **LI 4.**

   • **Stroke** from the elbow to the fingertips.

2. **Ear points:** wrist, shen men, sympathetic, liver.

Diet

- Avoid shellfish.

- Avoid cold and raw foods and iced drinks.

- Avoid greasy, fatty foods.

- Cut down on sour foods.

WRIST—CARPAL TUNNEL SYNDROME

Carpal tunnel syndrome is a common ailment that affects not only office workers who use computers, but anyone who repetitively grips, twists the wrist, or otherwise contracts the flexor muscles of the forearm and wrist. The carpal tunnel is a narrow area of the wrist through which the tendons of the fingers pass. If these tendons are used improperly or overused, they become inflamed. This causes fluid to build up in the tendon sheath. This swelling can narrow the tunnel, creating pressure on the median nerve, which also passes through this area. The result is pain and weakness of the forearm and hand. Usually, pain follows the pathway of the median nerve, going down the center of the forearm into the palm and middle and ring fingers.

Carpal tunnel syndrome is so prevalent in the public consciousness that other kinds of wrist pain are misdiagnosed as carpal tunnel syndrome. Rest and wrist braces can be useful initially, but Chinese medicine sees carpal tunnel syndrome as not only an overuse, but a misuse of the tendons and muscles of the arm and wrist. Tendons and muscles are not meant to be used independently, as in clicking a mouse when using the computer. Tendons and muscles are meant to be used in groups that contract and relax at the proper time, with the motion initiated from the spine or the center of the body. Therefore, rehabilitation must at some point involve exercises that reprogram the body's neuromuscular connections so that the arm is being used properly. Exercises like the **Daily Dozen** (chapter 5) and the **Eight Brocade Plus** (chapter 6) are invaluable in this kind of retraining and reintegration.

First Aid

1. Massage the wrist and forearm with **trauma liniment** (chapter 10).

2. Apply **san huang san** mixed with egg whites to the wrist, or use **Wu Yang pain-relieving plaster** (chapter 11).

3. Take two **trauma pills** a day for 2–3 days or **Reninall K** for 3–4 days (chapter 15).

4. Gently press **P 6** and the **heel pain point** on the palm of the hand (chapter 13) to help reduce pain and swelling.

5. Rest the arm and if necessary wear a brace to prevent further inflammation.

6. Avoid icing the wrist.

Follow-up Treatment

Once swelling and heat and redness (inflammation) are gone or significantly reduced:

1. Stop using the brace and begin to do exercises.

2. Massage **tendon lotion** or **U-I oil** (chapter 10) into the wrist several times a day

3. Soak the wrist in the **tendon-relaxing soak** (chapter 12) twice a day for 10 days.

Exercises

1. Do the **Daily Dozen** (chapter 5), especially **Arm Rotation, Elbow Rotation,** and **Pulling Nine Oxen.**

2. Do the **Eight Brocade Plus** (chapter 6), especially **Drawing the Bow to Shoot the Eagle,** the **Black Dragon Enters the Cave,** and **Embracing the Moon.**

3. Massage the meridians of the arms. Do exercise 11 of the **health preservation exercises** (chapter 7).

4. Practice the posture of holding a ball in front of the neck (see "Finger—Jammed").

Acupoints and Massage

1. Gently press **P 6** and the **heel pain point** on the palm several times a day to relieve pain and inflammation.

2. Massage treatment:

- Press **LI 11, LI 10, LI 4,** and **LU 6.**

- **Grasp** the muscles of the forearm from the elbow to the wrist.

- **Circular press** the tender areas of the wrist.

- **Stroke** from the elbow to the fingertips.

3. **Ear points:** wrist, shen men, sympathetic, liver.

Diet

- Avoid shellfish.

- Avoid cold and raw foods and iced drinks.

- Avoid greasy, fatty foods.

- Cut down on sour foods.

CHINESE SPORTS MEDICINE
FIRST-AID KIT

1 bottle	trauma liniment
6–8	trauma pills
1 package	yunnan paiyao powder
1 package	yunnan paiyao capsules
1 tube	Ching Wan Hung burn ointment
2–3	cups for cupping—different sizes
10	lancets for bleeding
1 pair	tweezers—to put ear seeds or pellets on ear points; to remove splinters
1 bottle	black ghost oil
1 quart-size plastic bag	san huang san (powder)
1 box	yunnan paiyao plaster
1 can	Wu Yang pain-relieving plasters
1 can	701 plasters
1 box	pellets or seeds, to stimulate ear points
2	moxa poles

6–10 rolls	rolled gauze
15–20	gauze pads
2–3	elastic bandages
2–3	self-adhering elastic bandages
1 pair	scissors—to cut bandages, tape, and gauze
30–40	Band-Aids—various sizes
1	triangular bandage—makes a sling for injured arm or collarbone
1	unbreakable plastic bottle—to dispose of lancets

WHERE TO BUY CHINESE HERBS AND EQUIPMENT

There are many stores where herbs, equipment, and other supplies mentioned in this book can be purchased. I have listed Chinese herb stores that will ship herbs and require only the romanized names of the herbs that are listed in this book. In general, calling ahead before faxing one of these shops is a good idea. Also, remember that if the herbs need to be ground, this will entail an additional fee.

CHINESE HERB STORES

There are many fine Chinese herb stores in North America. I have selected for this list herb stores that I know personally or have been recommended to me by other practitioners of Chinese medicine. All carry a fairly complete selection of Chinese herbs as well as some of the equipment mentioned in his book, such as cups and ear beads and seeds, and are willing to grind and ship herbs anywhere. Each store also has English speakers on staff.

CHINA HERB CO.
165 W. Queen Lane
Philadelphia, PA 19144
Tel: (215) 843-5864
Fax: (215) 849-3338
(800) 221-4372

FAR EAST GINSENG HERBS AND TEA
33162 Dequindre Rd.
Sterling Heights, MI 48310
Tel: (586) 977-0202
Fax: (586) 977-6688
www.fareastginseng.com

GEN MIN
2841 University Ave.
San Diego, CA 92104
Tel: (619) 297-0446
Fax: (619) 297-2628

KAM WO HERB & TEA
211 Grand St.
New York, NY 10013
Tel: (212) 966-6370
     (212) 925-2338
Fax: (212) 226-4717
www.kamwo.com

LIN SISTER HERB SHOP INC.
4 Bowery
New York, NY 10013
Tel: (212) 962-5417
     (212) 962-0477
Fax: (212) 587-8826
linsisterherbs@aol.com

EAST WEST HERB SHOP
3 Neals Yard
Covent Garden, London WC2H 9DP
Tel: 0171-3791312
Fax: 0171-3794414

EAST WEST HERBS LTD.
Langston Priory Mews
Kingham, Oxfordshire OX7 6UP
Tel: 01608-658862
Fax: 01608-658816

OTHER SUPPLIERS

HICKEY CHEMISTS
(800) 724-5566 (eastern standard time)
Monday–Friday 8:30 a.m. to 7:00 p.m.
Saturday 10:00 a.m. to 6:00 p.m.
info@hickeychemists.com
www.hickeychemists.com

Four Locations:

1. 434 Sixth Ave.
(corner of 10th St.)
New York, NY 10011
Tel: (212) 777-0008
Fax: (212) 777-0930

2. 1258 Third Ave.
(between 72nd and 73rd Sts.)
New York, NY 10021
Tel: (212) 744-5944
Fax: (212) 744-5988

3. 888 Second Ave.
(between 47th and 48th Sts.)
New York, NY 10017
Tel: (212) 223-6333
Fax: (212) 980-1533

4. 1645A Jericho Turnpike
(two blocks east of New Hyde Park Rd.)
New Hyde Park, NY 11040
Tel: (800) 724-5566
Fax: (516) 616-5770

Hickey Chemists carries many herbal products, including Resinall K (Health Concerns) and Liquid Liver Extract (Enzymatic Therapy).

K. S. CHOI CORP.
3932 Wilshire Blvd. #300
Los Angeles, CA 90010
Tel: (213) 380-9940
Fax: (213) 380-9951
www.acuzone.com

OMS MEDICAL SUPPLIES, INC.
1950 Washington St.
Braintree, MA 02184
(781) 331-3370
Toll-free orders: (800) 323-1839
Fax: (781) 335-5779
www.omsmedical.com

One of the oldest and largest suppliers of equipment for Eastern medicine—moxa equipment, ear seeds and beads, cupping sets, and so on.

ORIENTAL HERB COMPANY
3202 North West Highway #168
Cary, IL 60013
Tel: (800) 635-HERB
Fax: (847) 639-7199
www.orientalherb.com

This company carries many liniments made specifically for martial arts training and sports injuries, including Chinese Massage Oil.

YCY CHINESE MEDICINE & HEALTH CARE CENTER
USA toll-free: (866) 685-1871
Canada and international: (604) 685-1871
Fax: (604) 676-0192
sales@ycyhealth.com

REDWING BOOK CO.
44 Linden St.
Brookline, MA 02445
Tel: (800) 873-3946
Fax: (617) 738-4620
orders@redwingbooks.com
www.redwingbooks.com

202 Bendix Dr.
Taos, NM 87571
Tel: (505) 758-7768
Fax: (505) 758-7768

Redwing is one of the largest distributors of books on Eastern medicine and related subjects in the United States.

WILLNER CHEMISTS
100 Park Ave.
New York, NY 10017
Tel: (800) 633-1106 (orders)
Tel: (212) 682-2817
Fax: (212) 682-6192

253 Broadway
New York, NY 10007
Tel: (212) 791-0505
Fax: (212) 791-1201

2900 Peachtree Rd., N.E.
Atlanta, GA 30305
Tel: (404) 266-9115
    (866) 266-3746
Fax: (404) 237-6698
www.willner.com
cutserv@willner.com

*Willner Chemists carries many herbal products, including Resinall K
(Health Concerns) and Liquid Liver Extract (Enzymatic Therapy).*

INDEX

ABOUT THE AUTHOR

Tom Bisio is a world-renowned martial artist who has practiced and taught martial arts for the last twenty-eight years in the United States and the Far East. He is also a licensed practitioner of Chinese medicine, acupuncture, and herbalism. During numerous trips to China and Southeast Asia, he studied both medicine and martial arts with many different masters. He learned to treat his own injuries and tested the effectiveness of his formulas while competing in full-contact stick fighting and open kung fu tournaments in New York's Chinatown.

With a B.A. from Columbia University in East Asian Studies and courses in exercise physiology, Tom has extensive experience as a trainer at the most elite fitness centers in New York City, where he worked closely with sports trainers, physical therapists, and movement therapists. His diverse and unique background in both Western and Eastern approaches to healing has helped him effectively create and implement rehabilitation programs for injured athletes.

Currently, Tom heads a clinic that specializes in trauma and sports injuries and conducts seminars throughout the country teaching Chinese sports medicine to thousands of people. He is the former president of North American Tang Shou Tao, a national kung fu association.